P◻CKET PIMPED

INTERNAL MEDICINE

Donevan R. Westerveld, MD

Zachary M. V. Sherman, MD

© 2021 Pocket Pimped, LLC
www.PocketPimped.com
ISBN: 978-1-7343287-1-4

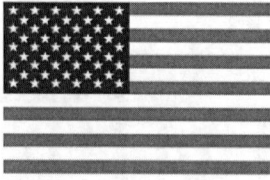

Printed in the United States of America

NOTICE

Editors and Contributors

Kirana Gudi, MD

Program Director, Weill Cornell Medicine/
NewYork Presbyterian Internal Medicine Residency
Vice Chair of Education, Weill Department of Medicine
Assistant Professor of Medicine, Division of PCCM
Weill Cornell Medicine
New York, NY

Uday S. Nori, MD, FASN, FNKF

Clinical Associate Professor of Medicine
Program Director, Nephrology Fellowship
The Ohio State University Wexner Medical Center
Columbus, OH

Carl V. Crawford, MD

Assistant Professor of Clinical Medicine
Program Director of the Gastroenterology and
Hepatology Fellowship Program
Division of Gastroenterology & Hepatology –
Department of Medicine
Weill Cornell Medicine/NewYork Presbyterian Hospital
New York, NY

Dana J. Lukin, MD, PhD, FACG

Clinical Director of Translational Research
Jill Roberts Center for Inflammatory Bowel Disease
Associate Professor of Clinical Medicine
Program Director, Advanced Fellowship in IBD
Weill Cornell Medicine/NewYork Presbyterian Hospital
New York, NY

Editors and Contributors

Amir Ahmadi, MD, FRCPC, FACC, FSCCT
Assistant Professor of Medicine
Icahn School of Medicine at Mount Sinai
Director, Inpatient Cardiology
Co-Director, Cardiac Intensive Care Unit
Associate Program Director, Cardiology Fellowship
Training Program
Mount Sinai Heart at Morningside
New York, NY

David Wan, MD
Assistant Professor of Medicine
Assistant Program Director of the Gastroenterology and
Hepatology Fellowship Program
Division of Gastroenterology & Hepatology –
Department of Medicine
Weill Cornell Medicine/NewYork Presbyterian Hospital
New York, NY

Dianne Goede, MD
Assistant Professor
Associate Chief for Quality and Patient Safety
Department of Medicine, Division of Internal Medicine
University of Florida College of Medicine
Gainesville, FL

Alexander Merkler, MD, MS
Assistant Professor of Neurology
Weill Cornell Medicine/NewYork Presbyterian Hospital
New York, NY

Editors and Contributors

Margaret C. Lo, MD

Professor of Medicine
Associate Program Director, UF Internal
Medicine Residency Program
Program Co-Director, VA Chief Residency in
Quality Safety
Director, UF Primary Care Track
Department of Medicine, Division of Internal Medicine
University of Florida College of Medicine
Gainesville, FL

Arun B. Jesudian, MD

Assistant Professor of Medicine
Director of Inpatient Liver Services
Weill Cornell Medicine/NewYork Presbyterian Hospital
Division of Gastroenterology and Hepatology
Center for Liver Disease and Transplantation
New York, NY

Rebecca Beyth, MD, MSc

Professor of Medicine
Associate Program Director, UF Internal
Medicine Residency Program
Associate Director, GRECC-Clinical Innovation
Director, VA CRQS Program
Department of Medicine, Division of Internal Medicine
University of Florida College of Medicine
Gainesville, FL

David Fernandez, MD, PhD

Assistant Attending Physician, Hospital for Special Surgery
Assistant Attending Physician, Weill Cornell Medicine
New York, NY

Editors and Contributors

Adrian Majid, MD
Assistant Professor of Medicine
Section of Hospital Medicine
Division of General Internal Medicine
Weill Cornell Medicine
New York, NY

Amy J. Sheer MD, MPH
Assistant Professor of Medicine
Department of Medicine, Division of Internal Medicine
University of Florida College of Medicine
Gainesville, FL

Medha Barbhaiya MD, MPH
Assistant Attending Physician, Hospital for Special Surgery
Assistant Professor of Medicine and
Population Health Sciences,
Weill Cornell Medicine
New York, NY

Ghaith Abu-Zeinah, MD
Instructor in Medicine
Division of Hematology and Oncology
Weill Cornell Medicine
New York, NY

Aaron S. Fisher, DO
Clinical Assistant Professor of Internal Medicine
University of Michigan
Ann Arbor, MI

Editors and Contributors

Rocio Salas-Whalen, MD
Endocrinology, Diabetes & Obesity
Owner of New York Endocrinology
Clinical Instructor at NYU Langone Medical Center
New York, NY

Joseph A. Daibes, DO
Chief Cardiology Fellow
Icahn School of Medicine at Mount Sinai
Mount Sinai Heart at Morningside
Mount Sinai West
James J. Peters VA Medical Center
New York, NY

Jori Kaplan, MD
Hematology/Oncology Fellow
H. Lee Moffitt Cancer Center & Research Institute
Tampa, FL

Nina Massad, MD
Neurocritical Care Fellow
Weill Cornell Medicine/Columbia University/
NewYork Presbyterian
New York, NY

This book is dedicated to my wife Julie without whom none of my success would have been possible. You are the heart of our family and you never cease to amaze me. To my children, Dominic and Annabelle, you are the loves of my life and the reason I rush home.

-Donevan

For my wife Suzanne - without your unconditional love and support I would not be who I am, or where I am today. And for my daughters, Julia and Rebecca - you both are the bright light I look forward to at the end of a long day.

-Zachary

x

Contents

- Cardiovascular
- Metabolic & Endocrine
- Urogenital
- Musculoskeletal
- Miscellaneous

Hematology   143

Infectious Disease — 163

Oncology 219

Pulmonology 231

Preface

The concept of pimping, or asking questions to test one's knowledge, is a long-time tradition that provides perspective to an individual's preparedness and understanding of a topic. In Internal Medicine, each case or disease process has a group of questions that are predictably asked. It was the recognition of this pattern that sparked the beginning of *Pocket Pimped*. This book is a collection of common pimp questions that we, as residents, fellows, and attendings either ask or have been asked. We hope that the reader may use this book as a resource to be better prepared and to guide their studies as they begin to decipher what is important in their journey to becoming a better physician. The authors wish the readers all the best in their pursuit.

GENERAL INTERNAL MEDICINE

Screening

All recommendations per 2020 USPSTF guidelines

Breast Cancer

1. At what age is breast cancer screening with mammography recommended in women of average risk?

> ➢ 50-74 years old

Cervical Cancer & HPV

2. At what age should women undergo cervical cancer screening?

> ➢ 21-65 years old

3. What are the two primary tests used for cervical cancer screening?

> ➢ Pap smear for cervical cytology and HPV DNA

4. At what age should HPV DNA testing be considered for cervical cancer screening?

> ➢ ≥30 years old

5. What is the screening interval for Pap smears in women 21-29 years old? Women 30-65 years old?

> ➢ 21-29 years old: Every 3 years for Pap smear only with a normal prior result
> ➢ 30-69 years old: Every 5 years for Pap smear plus HPV DNA negative results

Abdominal Aortic Aneurysm (AAA)

6. In what patient population is a one-time abdominal aortic aneurysm screening with abdominal ultrasound recommended?

➤ Men 65-75 years old who have ever smoked

Diabetes

7. In what patient population is type 2 diabetes mellitus screening recommended?

➤ Adults 40-70 years old who are overweight or obese

Colorectal Cancer

8. When should colorectal screening be initiated in the average risk patient?

➤ 50 years old and continue until 75 years old

Sexually Transmitted Infections (STIs)

9. When should average risk patients be screened for HIV?

➤ 15-65 years old and all pregnant women

10. How often should high risk individuals (ie. men who have sex with men, IV drug users) be screened for HIV?

➤ Consider annually

11. What patient population should be screened for chlamydia and gonorrhea?

➤ Any sexually active woman ≤24 years old
➤ Women >24 years old who are at increased risk for infection

12. The USPSTF recommends screening for hepatitis C virus (HCV) infection for what age group of patients?

➤ Adults 18-79 years old

Lung Cancer

13. What patient population should undergo annual screening for lung cancer with low dose computed tomography?

> ➤ Adults 55-80 years old who have at least a 20 pack-year smoking history, who currently smoke or who have quit within the past 15 years

Osteopenia & Osteoporosis

14. What is the definition based upon T-score of osteopenia? Osteoporosis? Fragility fracture?

> ➤ Osteopenia: DEXA T-score of -1.0 to -2.4
> ➤ Osteoporosis: DEXA T-score of ≤-2.5
> ➤ Fragility fracture: A fracture that results from a fall from standing height or lower

15. What tool can be used to estimate the 10-year probability of a hip fracture or other major osteoporotic fracture in a patient untreated for osteoporosis?

> ➤ Fracture Risk Assessment Tool (FRAX tool)
>> ▪ Used in the patients between the 40-90 years old

16. When should women be screened for osteoporosis with a DEXA scan?

> ➤ Women ≥65 years old
> ➤ Postmenopausal women <65 years old with high-risk factors for osteoporosis as determined by a formal clinical risk assessment tool

- Risk factors: Glucocorticoid therapy, low body weight, current cigarette smoking, family history of hip fractures, alcohol use

Prostate Cancer

17. When is prostate cancer screening indicated?
    - For men 55-69 years old
      - However, the decision should be based on shared decision making with the patient as there are no societal recommendations for hard set indications for screening

Dyslipidemia

18. How often should patients be screened for dyslipidemia?
    - Optimal interval for screening is uncertain
    - Reasonable options include every 5 years (shorter for people who have lipid levels close to those warranting therapy, and longer intervals for those not at increased risk with repeatedly normal lipid levels)
    - An age at which to stop screening has not been established

Biostats

19. What is a cross-sectional study?
    - An observational study that evaluates the relationship between an outcome and intervention at a single point in time

20. How do positive likelihood ratios of 2, 5, and 10 change the post-test probability of a disease?
  ➢ They increase the post-test probability of a disease by 15%, 30%, and 45%, respectively

21. What is lead-time bias?
  ➢ Overestimation of the survival time from a screening test detecting a disease earlier during its preclinical phase when there is occult disease (opposed to later when there is overt disease)
  ➢ Simply reflects the earlier diagnosis, but the overall survival time is unchanged

22. What does the sensitivity of a test indicate?
  ➢ True positive rate

23. What does the specificity of a test indicate?
  ➢ True negative rate

24. Do positive and negative predictive values vary depending on the prevalence of a disease?
  ➢ Yes

25. Do sensitive and specificity vary depending on the prevalence of a disease?
  ➢ No

26. In what type of study design are odds ratios typically reported?
  ➢ Case control studies

27. In what type of study design are relative risks typically reported?
  ➢ Cohort studies and clinical trials

28. How do you calculate the relative risk reduction (RRR)?

➢ RRR = (control event rate – experimental event rate)/control event rate

➢ RRR = 1 - relative risk

29. How do you calculate the number needed to treat?

➢ NNT = 1/absolute risk reduction

30. What is the incidence rate?

➢ Number of new cases during a specified period of time divided by the number of people at risk

31. What is the prevalence rate?

➢ Number of existing cases at a point in time divided by total number of people in the population

32. What is a type I error?

➢ Incorrectly rejecting the null hypothesis (false positive error)

33. What is a type II error?

➢ Incorrectly accepting the null hypothesis (false negative error)

Preventative Health & Vaccinations

Live Attenuated Vaccines

34. What are common live attenuated vaccines that should be avoided in immunocompromised patients?

➢ Varicella

➢ Measles, mumps, rubella (MMR)

➢ Live attenuated influenza vaccine

Tetanus

35. What two factors help determine tetanus prophylaxis?

> ➤ Wound site: Determine if it is (a) clean or a minor wound, or (b) dirty or severe or "all other" wounds
>
> ➤ Tetanus toxoid administration history: Determine if the patient has had (a) ≥3 tetanus toxoid doses, or (b) if the patient is unimmunized, uncertain, or <3 tetanus toxoid doses

36. When do you administer tetanus toxoid containing vaccine with or without tetanus immunoglobulins?

> ➤ ≥3 lifetime tetanus toxoid doses
>> ▪ Clean or minor wound: Tetanus toxoid vaccine only if the last dose was ≥10 years prior
>> ▪ Dirty or severe or "all other" wounds: Tetanus toxoid vaccine only if the last dose was ≥5 years prior
>
> ➤ Unimmunized, uncertain, or <3 tetanus toxoid lifetime doses
>> ▪ Clean or minor wound: Tetanus toxoid containing vaccine only
>> ▪ Dirty or severe or "all other" wounds: Tetanus toxoid containing vaccine AND tetanus immunoglobulins
>
> ➤ Persons who have HIV or are severely immunocompromised with a contaminated wound should receive human tetanus

immunoglobin regardless of tetanus vaccination history

37. What are the routine tetanus, diphtheria, and pertussis (Tdap) vaccination recommendations in immunocompetent patients?

> ➤ All pregnant women between 27-36 weeks gestation for EVERY pregnancy
> ➤ Tetanus and diphtheria toxin (Td) booster every 10 years for all adults with a one-time Tdap vaccine in lieu of Td

Human Papillomavirus (HPV)

38. When should the HPV vaccine be administered in immunocompetent individuals?

> ➤ Men and women 11-12 years old (may be initiated as early as 9 years old)
> - If not obtained by 12 years old, vaccine may be given up to 26 years old
> - May consider vaccine up to 46 years old in patients that may benefit

39. What are the indications for a two-dose and three-dose schedule for HPV vaccination?

> ➤ Two-dose schedule: Recommended for patients that receive their first dose prior to their 15th birthday, and the second dose 6-12 months after the first dose
> ➤ Three-dose schedule: Recommended for patients who get the first dose on or after their 15th birthday, or (2) have certain immunocompromised conditions, or (3) if a

second dose was administered before a 5-month
interval from the first dose

40. Should you restart the HPV vaccination series if a
patient misses a follow-up dose?

  ➢ No, continue without restarting the series

Meningitis

41. What is the routine vaccination recommendation
for the meningococcal conjugate vaccine in
immunocompetent adolescents and adults?

  ➢ Adolescents: All 11-12 year-olds should receive a
    meningococcal conjugate vaccine with a booster
    dose at 16 years old

    ▪ Serogroup B meningococcal vaccine is
      recommended for patients ≥10 years old if at
      increased risk of meningococcal disease

  ➢ Adults: College students living in dormitories,
    military recruits, exposed persons, asplenia or
    complement component deficiencies, and travels
    to endemic areas

42. What are the recommendations for vaccination
with serogroup B meningococcal vaccine?

  ➢ Adolescent and adults preferably 16-18 years old
    may receive this vaccine and should if they are at
    increased risk of medical conditions (ie. asplenia
    or complement component deficiencies) or
    environmental outbreaks (ie. college students
    living in dormitories, military recruits, exposed
    persons, and travel to endemic areas)

Shingles

43. What is recommended age for vaccination of the Zoster recombinant (Shingrix) vaccine?

> ➤ Zoster recombinant: A recombinant vaccine in use since 2017 and is now the preferred shingles vaccine by the CDC
>> ▪ Adults ≥50 years old should receive two doses spaced 2-6 months apart

Pneumonia

44. What are the two types of pneumococcal vaccines available in the United States?

> ➤ Pneumococcal conjugate vaccine (PCV13; Prevnar)
> ➤ Pneumococcal polysaccharide vaccine (PPSV23; Pneumovax)

45. What is the routine vaccine administration schedule for the pneumococcal vaccine?

> ➤ In patients 19-64 years old with a history of diabetes, alcoholism, cigarette smoking, chronic heart (excluding hypertension), lung, or liver disease: PPSV23 alone should be administered
>> ▪ At age 65 these individuals should then receive PCV13 followed by another dose of PPSV23 at least 1 year from prior PCV13
> ➤ Patients 19-64 years old who are immunocompromised (ie. HIV, malignancy, nephrotic syndrome, solid organ transplant), CSF leaks, cochlear implants, sickle cell disease, iatrogenic immunosuppressive, asplenism, or

CKD should receive sequential vaccination with
PCV13 followed by PPSV23 8 weeks apart
- A subsequent dose of PPSV23 should be given
  at least 5 years thereafter (or at 65 years old)

Cardiovascular

46. What is the most appropriate pharmacologic
therapy for primary prevention of atherosclerotic
cardiovascular disease (ASCVD) and colorectal cancer
in adults?
   ➤ Daily low dose (81 mg) aspirin

47. What are the indications for initiating statin therapy
for primary prevention of cardiovascular disease?
   ➤ Adults 40-75 years old without a history of CVD
     who have ≥1 CVD risk factors (ie. HTN,
     tobacco use, diabetes) and calculated 10-year risk
     of cardiovascular events of ≥10%

48. Which lab tests should be ordered before initiation
of a statin?
   ➤ Liver functions test and lipid panel

Obesity

49. What BMI range is defined as underweight?
Normal weight? Overweight? Obese class I? Obese
class II? Obese class III?
   ➤ Underweight: <18.5 kg/m^2
   ➤ Normal weight: ≥18.5 to 24.9 kg/m^2
   ➤ Overweight: ≥25.0 to 29.9 kg/m^2
   ➤ Obese class I: 30.0 to 34.9 kg/m^2
   ➤ Obese class II: 35.0 to 39.9 kg/m^2

➢ Obese class III: ≥ 40 kg/m^2

50. When should patients be referred for bariatric surgery?

➢ Patients who have failed to lose weight despite lifestyle modification with a BMI ≥ 40 or BMI ≥ 35 with obesity-related comorbidities such as type 2 diabetes mellitus, CAD, osteoarthritis, or obstructive sleep apnea

51. What are the three main types of bariatric surgery?

➢ Roux-en-Y gastric bypass surgery, sleeve gastrectomy, and gastric banding

52. Long-term post-bariatric surgical care should focus on what deficiencies?

➢ Nutritional deficiencies such as fat-soluble vitamins, iron, folate, calcium, copper, zinc, and thiamine

➢ Patients who have undergone bariatric surgery require lifelong vitamin and mineral replacement

53. What patient population is a candidate for pharmacological weight loss therapy?

➢ Patients with a BMI ≥ 30, or a BMI ≥ 27 with weight-related comorbidities who have failed comprehensive lifestyle modifications

54. What are the three most commonly prescribed pharmacological options for the treatment of obesity?

➢ Orlistat, GLP-1 receptor agonist (ie. Liraglutide), phentermine-topiramate

55. What are the primary side effects of Orlistat therapy?

> Gastrointestinal upset including flatus, fecal incontinence, and borborygmi
  - Avoid in patients with chronic diarrhea
> Hypoglycemia in diabetic patients

56. What are the primary side effects of GLP-1 receptor agonists?

> Diarrhea, hypoglycemia (in combination of sulfonylurea), nausea, vomiting, tachycardia, and injection site reaction

57. What are the primary side effects of phentermine-topiramate?

> Dry mouth, constipation, and paresthesias
  - Avoid phentermine in those with cardiovascular disease (may cause tachycardia), uncontrolled hypertension, uncontrolled anxiety, active substance abuse disorder, pregnancy or breastfeeding
  - Avoid topiramate in those with a history of renal stones, pregnancy, breast feeding, or planning for pregnancy

58. What pharmacologic medication for obesity was removed from the market due to concerns of increased risk of malignancy?

> Lorcaserin

Mental Health

59. What are the two most common mental health conditions in patients seen in primary care?

> Anxiety and depression

60. What mental health disorder may frequently present as depression but should be ruled out prior to initiating antidepressants?

> Bipolar disorder
> - Should be ruled out prior to initiating antidepressants as treatment with antidepressants alone may increase the risk of mania and hypomania

61. What pre-screening questionnaire is used for depression? If positive, which more detailed screening questionnaire is used?

> Pre-screening: Patient Health Questionnaire 2 (PHQ-2)
> - Has a sensitivity and specificity of 95% and 57%, respectively
> More detailed: Patient Health Questionnaire 9 (PHQ-9)

62. What two questions comprise the PHQ-2?

> During the last month, have you often been bothered by feeling down, depressed, or hopeless?
> During the last month, have you often been bothered by having little interest or pleasure in doing things?

63. What constitutes a positive screening on the PHQ-2?

> A single yes response, or a score ≥3, indicates possible clinical significance for depression and should be further investigated

64. What are risk factors for depression?

➢ Female sex, alcohol dependence, personal or family history of depression, recent childbirth, recent stressful event

65. What is an important distinguishing factor between the patient health questionnaire 9 (PHQ-9) and the DSM-5 criteria for major depression?

➢ PHQ-9 also measures disease severity

66. What are the PHQ-9 disease severity score ranges?

➢ Non-depressed: 0-4

➢ Minor depression: 5-9

➢ Mild depression: 10-14

➢ Moderately severe depression: 15-19

➢ Severe depression: 20-27

67. What is a neurologic adverse effect of bupropion?

➢ Lowers the seizure threshold

68. What are two clinically useful adverse effects of mirtazapine?

➢ Somnolence and increased appetite

69. What are common gastrointestinal adverse effect of sertraline?

➢ Higher incidence of diarrhea, nausea, and dry mouth (xerostomia)

70. First generation antidepressants such as amitriptyline and desipramine are contraindicated for use with what other class of medications?

➢ Monoamine oxidase inhibitors

71. What is the only SSRI with a class D rating for pregnancy?

➢ Paroxetine

72. What is first-line pharmacological therapy for anxiety disorder?
> SSRI

73. What are 3 common unwanted side effects of SSRIs?
> Sexual dysfunction, weight gain, agitation
  ▪ Sexual dysfunction is estimated to occur in up to 50% of patients taking SSRIs

74. How do you manage sexual dysfunction as a side effect of an SSRI?
> Either switch to another SSRI or switch to a non-SSRI such as bupropion that causes less sexual side effects

75. What is first-line pharmacologic treatment for premature ejaculation?
> SSRIs or SNRIs

76. What is the first-line treatment for social anxiety disorder?
> Cognitive-behavioral therapy or SSRI
> Do not prescribe benzodiazepines as first-line treatment

77. What symptoms must be present to diagnose panic disorder?
> An abrupt surge of intense fear or discomfort that reaches a peak within minutes and during which time ≥4 of the following occur:
  ▪ Palpitations, pounding heart, or accelerated heart rate
  ▪ Sweating
  ▪ Trembling or shaking

- Sensations of shortness of breath or smothering
- Feelings of choking
- Chest pain or discomfort
- Nausea or abdominal distress
- Feeling dizzy, unsteady, light-headed, or faint
- Chills or heat sensations
- Paresthesias (numbness or tingling sensations)
- Derealization (feelings of unreality) or depersonalization (being detached from oneself)
- Fear of losing control or "going crazy"
- Fear of dying

78. What is the treatment for panic disorder?
   ➢ Cognitive-behavioral therapy and SSRIs are first-line

79. What criteria must be met to diagnose binge eating disorder?
   ➢ ≥3 of the following occurring at least once weekly for a minimum of three months:
      - Consuming large amounts of food when not hungry
      - Abnormally rapid consumption
      - Eating alone due to embarrassment
      - Feeling guilty due to overconsumption
      - Eating until uncomfortably full

80. How can you distinguish between binge eating disorder (BED) and bulimia nervosa?

➢ While both include episodes of binge eating, BED lacks the compensatory behaviors to avoid weight gain

81. Which common antipsychotics are associated with causing prolonged QT intervals?

➢ Haloperidol, atypical>typical antipsychotics, lithium, tricyclic anti-depressants

Vitamin & Mineral Deficiencies

82. What vitamin deficiencies are associate with cognitive deficits and depression in chronic alcoholics?

➢ Folate
➢ Thiamine (Vitamin B1)

83. What vitamin deficiency commonly causes macrocytic anemia and intestinal malabsorption in chronic alcoholics?

➢ Folate

84. What mineral deficiency seen in post bariatric surgery patients can manifest with ataxia, neuropathy, cognitive deficits, and anemia?

➢ Copper which closely mimics a Vitamin B12 deficiency

85. What vitamin deficiency is associated with the triad of dermatitis (pellagra), diarrhea, and dementia?

➢ Niacin (Vitamin B3)
  ▪ Risk factors include alcoholism and bariatric weight loss surgery

86. What vitamin deficiency is associated with perifollicular hemorrhage, petechiae, and bruising?

➢ Vitamin C

19

87. What vitamin deficiency is associated with paresthesias, gait instability, psychiatric issues, and macrocytic anemia?

> Vitamin B12

88. What mineral excess is associated with neurologic symptoms, psychiatric symptoms, vision symptoms, and cirrhosis?

> Copper accumulation in the setting of Wilson's disease

89. What is the most common hematologic manifestation of Vitamin B12 deficiency?

> Megaloblastic or macrocytic anemia

90. Which fish tapeworm infection is classically associated with a Vitamin B12 deficiency?

> Diphyllobothrium latum
  - The tapeworm competes for the absorption of Vitamin B12

91. What autoimmune diseases are commonly associated with a Vitamin B12 deficiency?

> Pernicious anemia
> IBD

92. What water-soluble vitamin deficiency is associated with night blindness and loss of taste?

> Vitamin A
  - Commonly seen in post-bariatric surgery patients

93. What vitamin deficiency is associated with accelerated bone loss, secondary hyperparathyroidism, and increased risk of fractures?

> Vitamin D

94. What lab test measurement is used to evaluate Vitamin D sufficiency?

> 25-hydroxyvitamin D (calcidiol)

95. Testing for which metabolites distinguishes a diagnosis of Vitamin B12 deficiency from a folate deficiency?

> Methylmalonic acid (MMA) is elevated in Vitamin B12 deficiency and normal in folate deficiency

Primary Care

Pharyngitis & Sinusitis

96. What criteria is used to diagnose streptococcal pharyngitis?

> Centor criteria (one point each):
>   - **F**ever
>   - **A**bsence of cough
>   - **C**ervical lymphadenopathy (anterior)
>   - **E**xudates or swelling of the tonsils
>   - Remember: "**FACE**"

97. If using the Centor criteria for assessing the likelihood of S. pharyngitis, what number of points may warrant additional rapid strep testing?

> ≥3 points

98. What is the first line therapy for streptococcal pharyngitis?

> Penicillin V or Amoxicillin

99. What is the classic cardiac complication of late untreated streptococcal pharyngitis?

> Mitral valve stenosis

100. Which signs differentiate bacterial from viral rhinosinusitis?

> Bacterial rhinosinusitis: Symptoms lasting ≥10 days, double sickening, upper teeth pain, and unilateral maxillary sinus tenderness

> The majority of cases are viral (98%)

Headaches

101. What are the 4 major types of headaches?

> Frontal, migraine, cluster, tension

102. What are considered headache "danger signs" that require further workup?

> **S**ystemic symptoms including fever

> **N**eoplasm history

> **N**eurologic deficit (including decreased consciousness)

> **O**nset is sudden or abrupt

> **O**lder age (onset after age 50 years)

> **P**attern change or recent onset of new headache

> **P**ositional headache

> **P**recipitated by sneezing, coughing, or exercise

> **P**apilledema

> **P**rogressive headache and atypical presentations

> **P**regnancy or puerperium

> **P**ainful eye with autonomic features

> **P**ost-traumatic onset of headache

> **P**athology of the immune system such as HIV

> **P**ainkiller (analgesic) overuse (ie. medication overuse headache) or new drug headaches

  - Remember: "**SNNOOP10**"

103. What are the pharmacologic abortive therapies for migraine headaches?
> Mild-to-moderate symptoms: Oral NSAIDs, acetaminophen, triptans
> Severe symptoms: IV or IM dihydroergotamine, metoclopramide, ketorolac

104. What are the preventive therapies for migraine headaches?
> Amitriptyline, venlafaxine, beta blockers (ie. propranolol or metoprolol), topiramate

105. In a woman with migraines with aura, what medication is contraindicated due to the increased risk of stroke?
> Combined oral contraceptives

Fibromyalgia

106. What are the characteristic findings of fibromyalgia?
> Widespread pain or tenderness of at least 3 months, sleep disturbances, and fatigue in the absence of joint swelling

107. What are the treatment options for fibromyalgia?
> Nonpharmacologic therapies: Patient education acknowledging the disease and prognosis, exercise, good sleep hygiene, addressing associated comorbidities
> Pharmacologic therapies: Amitriptyline, duloxetine
▪ Opioids are **NEVER** the answer

Infections

108. What pharmacologic therapy has been shown to reduce the risk of acquiring HIV?

> Pre-exposure prophylaxis with tenofovir-emtricitabine combination therapy

109. What are the indications for treatment of asymptomatic bacteriuria?

> Pregnancy, urinary tract surgery/interventions

110. What are the indications for treatment of asymptomatic candiduria?

> Neutropenia, urinary tract surgery/interventions

111. What organism is the most common cause of cystitis?

> Escherichia coli

112. What are common signs and symptoms of a complicated urinary tract infection?

> Fever, costovertebral tenderness, systemic signs of infection, symptoms of illness, flank pain, pelvic or perineal pain in men

113. What are the common first line therapies for uncomplicated cellulitis?

> Cefalexin, bactrim, fosfomycin, nitrofurantoin

114. What are classic features of complicated cellulitis?

> Abscess seen on exam or ultrasound, deep wound infections including decubitus ulcers and necrotizing fasciitis, purulent drainage concerning for methicillin-resistant Staphylococcus aureus (MRSA) infection

115. What is the most common organism causing abscess formation?

> MRSA

116. What are appropriate oral antibiotic therapies for a patient with an abscess skin infection? What procedure should be performed for most abscesses?

> Trimethoprim-sulfamethoxazole, doxycycline, minocycline, clindamycin
> Incision and drainage (I&D)

117. What is the first line therapy for tinea pedis?

> Topical antifungal therapies such as azoles and allylamines such as terbinafine

118. What are the common signs and symptoms of epididymitis?

> Superior testicular pain to palpation, erythema, swelling of a hemiscrotum, and abdominal pain

119. What two organisms are the most common infectious causes of acute epididymitis in a patient <35 years old? Older men? What is the treatment of choice?

> <35 years old: Chlamydia trachomatis and Neisseria gonorrhoeae
>   ▪ Treatment includes ceftriaxone 250 mg intramuscular injection plus doxycycline 100 mg BID x 10 days
> Older men: Escherichia coli and Pseudomonas
>   ▪ Treatment includes Levofloxacin 500 mg once daily x 10 days

Osteopenia & Osteoporosis

120. What is the most common cause of osteoporosis in women? In men?

> Women: Estrogen deficiency

> Men: Testosterone deficiency

121. What are the indications of antiresorptive therapy?
> Osteoporosis
> History of fragility fracture
> Vertebral or hip fractures
> Osteopenia in the setting of high-risk factors including a FRAX score >3% for hip fracture or ≥20% for major osteoporotic fracture

122. Why must patients remain upright for 30 minutes following the administration of oral bisphosphonates?
> Risk of erosive esophagitis

Varicocele

123. What is the first line treatment for a symptomatic left sided varicocele?
> Analgesic agents with scrotal support

124. What imaging should be obtained in a patient with a right sided varicocele? Why?
> CT scan
> Because the gonadal vein directly empties into the IVC, right sided varicoceles may be associated with inferior vena cava obstruction from a tumor or thrombosis

Benign Prostate Hyperplasia (BPH)

125. What class of medications is first line treatment in patients with mild to moderate symptoms of BPH?
> Alpha adrenergic receptor antagonist

126. What two common adverse effects are associated with terazosin and doxazosin?

> Dizziness and hypotension

Trigeminal Neuralgia

127. What are the clinical features of trigeminal neuralgia?
> Triggered paroxysmal sharp and stabbing pain burst in the facial nerve distribution and pain restricted to the territory of one or more division of the trigeminal nerve

128. What side of the face is most commonly affected by trigeminal neuralgia?
> Right side

129. What is the first line therapy for trigeminal neuralgia?
> Carbamazepine or oxcarbazepine

Macular Degeneration

130. What are cardinal retinal features of early age-related macular degeneration?
> Yellowish deposits known as drusen and focal hypo- or hyperpigmentation

131. What are cardinal features of late-stage age related macular degeneration?
> Loss of outer retina and the development of abnormal vasculature in the macular retina

132. What pharmacotherapies can prevent progression from early to late age-related macular degeneration?
> Vitamin C and E, beta carotene, and zinc

Peripheral Artery Disease (PAD)

133. What is the preferred initial diagnostic test in a patient with symptomatic peripheral artery disease?

> ➢ Ankle brachial index (ABI)

134. How is the ABI calculated?

> ➢ Dividing the dorsalis pedis or posterior tibial systolic pressure (whichever is higher) by the higher of the left or right brachial systolic pressure

135. What ABI range is considered normal? When is exercise treadmill ABI testing indicated? What is an office-based alternative to exercise treadmill ABI?

> ➢ Normal: 0.91-1.3 mmHg
> ➢ In patients with normal or borderline ABI who have exertional related leg pain
> ➢ Office based: Plantar flexion ABI

Coronary Artery Disease (CAD)

136. What are modifiable coronary artery disease risk factors? Non-modifiable risk factors?

> ➢ Modifiable: Smoking, alcohol intake, hypertension, obesity, type 2 diabetes, physical activity/sedentary lifestyle, high fat diet
> ➢ Non-modifiable: Family history, age, sex, genetic predisposition

Lipids & Triglycerides

137. What are common medications that can cause dyslipidemia?

> Corticosteroids, progesterone, beta blockers,
thiazide diuretics, androgenic steroids, oral
estrogen, antipsychotics

138. What is the primary target in lipid lowering
therapy to prevent coronary artery disease?

> Low density lipoprotein cholesterol (LDL-C)

139. What class of medication is the best for lowering
triglycerides?

> Fibrates

140. What is the most effective class of drug to raise
high density lipoprotein (HDL) cholesterol levels?

> Niacin

141. What are contraindications for treatment with
ezetimibe?

> Liver disease or elevated liver enzymes

142. Which statin should be avoided in patients taking
coumadin?

> Rosuvastatin

143. Omega 3 fatty acids can raise the level of which
cholesterol?

> HDL

144. What are the most common adverse effects of
statin therapy?

> Myalgia, limb pain, diarrhea, dyspepsia,
arthralgia, elevated transaminases

Miscellaneous

145. What serum laboratory test is commonly
depressed in people with restless leg syndrome?

> Ferritin

146. How do you differentiate between venous and arterial ulcers?
> Venous: Classically medial foot, superficial, dull aching discomfort, irregular shape
> Arterial: Classically lateral foot, full thickness wound, punched out appearance, with smooth wound edges, painful

147. What are the three most common pharmacotherapies for smoking cessation?
> Varenicline, bupropion, nicotine replacement therapy

Travel Medicine

Air Travel Oxygen

148. When is supplemental in-flight oxygen therapy required for a patient during long airline flights?
> Patient with a baseline resting SpO_2 <92% or PaO_2 <60 mmHg
> Patient with SpO_2 <84% or PaO_2 <55 mmHg during six-minute walk test

149. Patients on what amount of supplemental oxygen requirement is advised against any air travel?
> When their oxygen requirement at rest is >4L/minute
  ▪ Airlines cannot ensure sufficient supplemental in-flight oxygen for these patients

150. For patients with chronic oxygen requirement ≤4L/min, how do you advise them to adjust their oxygen requirement while in-flight?

> Increase their oxygen by 1-2 L/minute over their baseline oxygen requirement during flight

Traveler's Diarrhea & Infections

151. List three common microorganisms associated with infectious outbreaks with cruise travel?

> Influenza, norovirus, legionella

152. What are 4 common organisms that cause travelers' diarrhea? Which is the most common organism?

> Enterotoxigenic Escherichia coli (ETEC): Most common
> Salmonella species
> Campylobacter jejuni
> Rotavirus

153. Travel to which areas carry high risk (>20%) of contracting travelers' diarrhea?

> South and Southeast Asia, Africa (except for South Africa), Central America, South America, and Mexico

154. How do you treat travelers' diarrhea?

> First line: Fluid replacement, either orally or IV
>   - Most important
> Symptomatic management (ie. bismuth or anti-motility agents such as loperamide)
> Antibiotics for severe cases only (ie. azithromycin (preferred for fever or dysentery), fluoroquinolones, rifaximin, rifamycin)

Yellow Fever

155. Th yellow fever vaccination should be administered to patients traveling to what continents? What type of vaccine is this?
> ➤ Africa and South America
> ➤ Live attenuated

Hepatitis

156. Travel to which locations hold high risk for acquiring hepatitis A virus?
> ➤ South America, Central America, Mexico, Sub-Saharan Africa, South Asia

157. What are the two types of hepatitis A vaccines available?
> ➤ Monovalent vaccines (ie. HAVRIX or VAQTA)
> ➤ Bivalent (hepatitis A & B) combination vaccines (ie. Twinrix)

158. What is the administration schedule for the monovalent hepatitis A vaccines?
> ➤ 1 dose at any time before travel and second dose given 6-12 months later

Typhoid Fever

159. What is the causative agent of typhoid fever? Who is at highest risk for acquiring this disease?
> ➤ Salmonella enterica serotype Typhi
> ➤ Long-term travelers to resource-limited areas and those traveling to Southern Asia

Cholera

160. What is the route of transmission of cholera? Who should be vaccinated?

> ➤ Fecal oral route
> ➤ Adults traveling to an area of active transmission as identified by CDC (cdc.gov/travel)

Zika & Malaria

161. What type of insect repellent is highly effective at repelling mosquitos?

> ➤ DEET based (N,N-Diethyl-meta-toluamide)

162. How long should men who recently traveled to Zika endemic areas use barrier protection during intercourse AFTER returning from travel?

> ➤ 6 months regardless of symptoms

163. What are common symptoms of malaria?

> ➤ Fever (most common), chills, headache, sweats, fatigue, nausea and vomiting, diffuse weakness, diffuse myalgia, pallor

164. What are 5 different strains of malaria parasites? Which are resistant to chloroquine in certain endemic areas?

> ➤ Plasmodium falciparum: Resistant
> ➤ Plasmodium vivax: Resistant
> ➤ Plasmodium malaria
> ➤ Plasmodium ovale
> ➤ Plasmodium knowlesi

165. What is the primary strain of plasmodium in the USA?

> ➤ Plasmodium falciparum

166. What areas are highly endemic to chloroquine-resistant P. falciparum?

> Southeast Asia, India, Oceania, Africa, South America

167. What antimalarial agents are effective chemoprophylaxis in chloroquine-resistant malaria?

> Mefloquine, atovaquone-proguanil, doxycycline, and tafenoquine

168. What is the dosing schedule of mefloquine as an antimalarial prophylactic agent?

> Weekly, starting ≥2 weeks prior to travel and continued for 4 weeks after departure from endemic area

Altitude & Mountain Sickness

169. What are three types of altitude illnesses? What are their symptoms?

> Acute mountain sickness (AMS)
>   - Mimics alcohol hangover (ie. mostly headache with associated fatigue, nausea, vomiting, lightheaded, restless sleep)
> High altitude cerebral edema
>   - Mostly encephalopathic symptoms (ie. abnormal gait, confusion, irritability, severe fatigue, drowsiness, impaired mentation)
> High altitude pulmonary edema
>   - Early symptoms: Low-grade fever, dry cough and dyspnea on exertion
>   - Late symptoms: Low-grade fever, productive pink frothy sputum, shortness of breath at rest

and exercise intolerance with difficulty walking uphill
- Can be easily mistaken for URI or normal altitude fatigue

170. What is the most commonly prescribed medication for acute mountain sickness prophylaxis?
  ➢ Acetazolamide

171. What are the indications and options for prophylaxis in acute mountain sickness (AMS)?
  ➢ Persons with a history of AMS or those ascending rapidly to high altitude (>500 meters in a day above 3000 meters)
    - Acetazolamide prophylaxis, although slow gradual ascent is recommended over chemoprophylaxis (ie. no more than 300 meters per day with day of rest and no ascent every third day)
  ➢ Persons with co-morbidities vulnerable to hypoxic conditions (ie. CAD, COPD, OSA, sickle cell disease)
    - Prophylactic oxygen therapy

Hypertension

172. What are the 4 blood pressure categories for adults per the American Heart Association?
  ➢ Normal: Systolic pressure <120 mmHg **AND** diastolic <80 mmHg
  ➢ Elevated blood pressure: Systolic pressure of 120-129 mmHg and diastolic <80 mmHg

> Stage I hypertension: Systolic pressure of 130-139 mmHg **OR** diastolic 80-89 mmHg
> Stage II hypertension: Systolic pressure 140 mmHg **OR** diastolic ≥90 mmHg

173. What are common secondary causes of hypertension?

> Obstructive sleep apnea (OSA), medications (ie. steroids, NSAIDs), chronic renal disease, endocrine disorders (ie. Cushing's, pheochromocytoma, primary aldosteronism, thyroid disorders)

174. What medications should patients with hypertension avoid if possible?

> Steroids (anabolic and corticosteroids), NSAIDs, oral contraceptives containing estrogens, decongestants (ie. pseudoephrine), SSRI antidepressants (ie. venlafaxine)

175. What are some signs and symptoms that suggest secondary hypertension?

> New onset hypertension in age <25 or >55 years old
> Drug resistant hypertension or long-standing-to-control hypertension
> Epigastric abdominal bruit
> Palpitations, sweating, flushing, diarrhea, and headache (ie. pheochromocytoma)
> Moon facies, dorsocervical fat pad (aka buffalo hump), abdominal striae

176. What is the blood pressure treatment goal for an individual <65 years old per the American Heart Association?

> ➤ <130/80 mmHg

177. What is the definition of white coat hypertension?

> ➤ Consistently elevated in-office blood pressure measurements with normal out-of-office blood pressure measurements that do not meet criteria for hypertension

178. How do you further evaluate a patient with white coat hypertension?

> ➤ 24-hour ambulatory blood pressure monitoring (ABPM) with self-monitored blood pressure measurements averaged over 1 week

179. When should you consider treating white coat hypertension?

> ➤ With a confirmed daytime ABPM of ≥135/85 mmHg

180. What is the definition of masked hypertension?

> ➤ Blood pressure measurements that are consistently elevated at home or out-of-office but does not meet criteria for hypertension with in-office blood pressure measurements

181. How do you further evaluate a patient with masked hypertension?

> ➤ Ambulatory self-monitored blood pressure measurement (SMBP) for 1 week
>   - If SMBP is elevated above goal that first week, then obtain 24-hour ambulatory blood pressure monitoring (ABPM)

182. What are the complications of long-standing uncontrolled hypertension?

> Heart failure (systolic and/or diastolic), ischemic heart disease, left ventricular hypertrophy, ischemic or hemorrhagic stroke, retinopathy, chronic kidney disease

183. What retinal changes are seen in long-standing hypertension?

> Arteriolar narrowing, arteriovenous compression, papilledema, retinal hemorrhages or exudates

184. What are the 4 classes of medications that may be used as first line therapy in the management of hypertension?

> Angiotensin converting enzyme inhibitors (ACEi)
> Angiotensin receptor blockers (ARB)
> Thiazide diuretics
> Long acting (dihydropyridine) calcium channel blockers

185. What is the definition of drug-resistant hypertension?

> ≥3 antihypertensives at maximum dose (one of which is a diuretic)

186. What is the first line therapy for a patient with hypertension and chronic kidney disease (CKD)?

> ACEi/ARB

187. What is the first line therapy for hypertension in African American patients without CKD?

➤ Dihydropyridine calcium channel blocker or thiazide diuretic

188. What is the dietary approach used to reduce systolic blood pressure?

➤ Dietary approach to stopping hypertension (DASH) as developed by the National Institute of Health (NIH) and recommended by United States Department of Agriculture (USDA)

189. How much of a reduction in systolic blood pressure can be achieved with the DASH diet?

➤ ~5.5 mmHg

190. How much does systolic blood pressure improve with every 1 kilogram of body weight lost?

➤ ~1 mmHg

191. What are the adverse side effects of ACEi?

➤ Cough, angioedema, hyperkalemia, hypotension

192. What are the adverse side effects of calcium channel blockers?

➤ Headache, edema, constipation, hypotension

193. What are the common complications of thiazide diuretics?

➤ Photosensitivity and electrolyte abnormalities (ie. hyponatremia, hypokalemia), acute kidney injury, gout flare, hypotension, dehydration, pancreatitis

194. What lab tests should be ordered in a patient with newly diagnosed hypertension?

➤ Hemoglobin, serum electrolytes, fasting glucose, creatinine, lipid panel, and urinalysis with microscopy

195. What antihypertensive agent can cause gynecomastia in men?

> Spironolactone

Women's Health

Menopause

196. What are appropriate indications for treatment of vasomotor symptoms of menopause?

> Hormone therapy is appropriate in patients ≤60 years old and within 10 years of menopause onset in patients with low risk of thromboembolic disease, stroke, coronary artery disease, and breast cancer

197. What are the hormone replacement treatment options for vasomotor symptoms of menopause?

> Estrogen-progesterone therapy

198. What is the pharmacologic management of postmenopausal genitourinary syndrome of menopause?

> Vaginal estrogen therapy

Infections

199. Are women with cervicitis due to chlamydia trachomatis (C. trachomatis) typically symptomatic or asymptomatic?

> Overwhelmingly asymptomatic

200. What is the preferred treatment of candida vulvovaginitis?

> Single dose of 150 mg oral fluconazole

201. What are the clinical features required for the diagnosis of bacterial vaginosis (BV)?

> 3 of 4 of the following clinical features are required:
>   - Vaginal pH >4.5
>   - Positive whiff-amine test
>   - Thin and homogenous vaginal discharge with fishy odor
>   - Clue cells that comprise at least 20% of all squamous cells on wet mount

202. What is the treatment for BV?

> - Oral metronidazole 500 mg BID for 7 days
> - Metronidazole gel 0.75%, one full applicator (5g) intravaginally once a day for 5 days
> - Clindamycin cream 2%, one full applicator (5g) intravaginally at bedtime for 7 days

203. What is the most common sexually transmitted infection worldwide?

> - Trichomonas vaginalis

204. The presence of what organism on a vaginal smear wet mount is diagnostic for trichomonas vaginalis?

> - Motile flagellated protozoa in a spinning or jerky motion

205. What is the typical range of pH in trichomonas vaginalis?

> - >4.5

206. What is the treatment of trichomoniasis for the patient and relevant sexual partners?

> - Single dose of 2 grams of oral metronidazole

➢ The sexual partner(s) should also be treated with the same regimen

➢ Retesting for trichomonas vaginalis in women within 3 months of treatment is also appropriate

207. What organisms commonly cause pelvic inflammatory disease (PID)?

➢ C. trachomatis and Neisseria gonorrhoeae (N. gonorrhoeae) ascending infections

208. What is the preferred outpatient treatment regimen for PID?

➢ One dose of IM cephalosporin and oral doxycycline x 14 days

209. What are the complications of chronic PID?

➢ Perihepatitis, ectopic pregnancy, tubo-ovarian abscess

Polycystic Ovarian Syndrome (PCOS)

210. What are common dermatologic features of polycystic ovarian syndrome (PCOS)?

➢ Hirsutism, acne, hyperhidrosis

211. What is a common metabolic manifestation of PCOS?

➢ Insulin resistance

212. What is the treatment of choice in women with androgen-excess features of PCOS?

➢ Combined oral contraceptives (COC)

213. What is the first line imaging study in patients with suspected PCOS?

➢ Transvaginal and abdominal ultrasound with doppler

Contraceptives & Dysmenorrhea

214. What duration and frequency of smoking is a contraindication to COC use?

> ➤ Age ≥35 years and smoking ≥15 cigarettes/day

215. What are contraindications to the use of combined oral contraceptives (COC)?

> ➤ Current breast cancer
> ➤ Migraine with aura
> ➤ Tobacco use as above
> ➤ Known ischemic heart disease
> ➤ History of CVA
> ➤ Uncontrolled hypertension
> ➤ Decompensated cirrhosis

216. What is the duration of therapy for a levonorgestrel IUD?

> ➤ 3-6 years

217. What is the typical length of therapy for a copper intrauterine device (IUD)?

> ➤ 10 years

218. Does the copper IUD cause anovulation or amenorrhea?

> ➤ No

219. What are common gynecological adverse effects of the levonorgestrel IUD?

> ➤ Abnormal uterine bleeding, menstrual irregularity, pelvic pain, vaginal itching

220. What is the first line non-hormonal pharmacologic therapy for primary dysmenorrhea?

> ➤ NSAIDs

General Internal Medicine

Mastalgia

221. What is cyclic mastalgia?
> Bilateral and diffuse breast pain that often radiates to axilla and worsening in the days prior to menstruation but then abates thereafter

222. What is the common presentation of non-cyclical mastalgia? What is the recommended evaluation?
> Unilateral breast pain lasting for several days not associated with menses
> Patients <30 years old should undergo targeted breast ultrasound
> Patients ≥30 years old should undergo targeted breast ultrasound and diagnostic mammography to evaluate for breast malignancy

223. How do you treat mastalgia?
> Primarily reassurance and education, a well-fitting bra, and management of stress or anxiety/depression
> Pharmacologic treatments include topical NSAIDs (mild symptoms), tamoxifen as first line and danazol as second line (moderate symptoms), and goserelin (severe refractory symptoms)

Miscellaneous

224. What is a common cause of an erythematous pruritic rash underneath the breast of a woman? What is the treatment?
> Cutaneous candidiasis
> Nystatin cream or powder

225. What are red flags or warning signs that a patient may be a victim of human trafficking?
> Hesitancy in answering questions regarding injuries, inconsistent or scripted history, fearfulness or nervous behavior and demeanor, unawareness of current location
> Multiple pregnancies, miscarriages, and recurrent or untreated sexually transmitted infections

226. What are the most common etiologies of heavy menstrual bleeding?
> Adenomyosis or uterine leiomyomas

227. What are the most common presenting symptoms of endometriosis?
> Dysmenorrhea, heavy menstrual bleeding, chronic abdominal/pelvic pain

228. How long should a couple attempt to conceive prior to undergoing an evaluation for infertility?
> Women ≤35 should undergo evaluation after trying to conceive for over 12 months
> Women >35 should undergo evaluation after 6 months of trying to conceive

229. What is the time frame to suspect a diagnosis of postpartum depression?
> Depression that begins within 12 months of delivery

230. What are the indications of genetic testing for BRCA mutation?
> Any of the following:
  ▪ Triple negative breast cancer ≤60 years old
  ▪ Male breast cancer

- Breast cancer at any age and a relative with breast cancer diagnosed ≤50 years old
- Breast cancer diagnosis ≤45 years old

231. What is the most common cause of dyspareunia in women ≤50 years old? >50 years old?

➢ ≤50 years old: Vulvodynia

➢ >50 years old: Urogenital atrophy

232. What palpable external genital lesion commonly causes unilateral vaginal swelling and pain?

➢ Bartholin cyst

233. What antihypertensive medications are absolute contraindications during pregnancy?

➢ Angiotensin receptor blocker (ARBs) and angiotensin converting enzyme inhibitors (ACEi)

234. What are the signs and symptoms of ovarian torsion?

➢ Acute onset pelvic pain with nausea and vomiting

Physical Exam Findings

Cardiovascular

235. What are Osler nodes?

➢ Tender subcutaneous violaceous nodules on the pads of fingers and toes which are distal vasculitic lesions caused by immunologic phenomena in infective endocarditis

- May also be seen on thenar and hypothenar eminences

236. What are Janeway lesions?

> Nontender erythematous macules on palms and soles which are vasculitic lesions seen in infective endocarditis

237. What are Roth spots?
> Hemorrhagic retinal lesions seen in infective endocarditis

238. What is de Musset's sign?
> Head-bobbing with each heartbeat seen in aortic insufficiency

239. What is Muller's sign?
> Systolic pulsations of the uvula seen in aortic insufficiency

240. What is the classic auscultatory murmur heard in aortic stenosis?
> Mid systolic crescendo-decrescendo at right upper sternal border

241. What is the classic auscultatory murmur heard in mitral valve stenosis?
> Low pitched mid diastolic rumble at the apex with an opening snap

242. What is the classic auscultatory murmur heard in aortic insufficiency?
> Early diastolic decrescendo murmur heard best at left upper sternal border

243. What is the classic auscultatory murmur heard in mitral valve regurgitation?
> High pitched holosystolic murmur heard at the apex

244. What is the classic auscultatory murmur heard in mitral valve prolapse?

➢ High pitched mid systolic click

245. What is the classic auscultatory murmur heard in tricuspid valve regurgitation?

➢ High pitched holosystolic murmur best heard over left lower sternal border

246. What is Beck's triad in the pericardial tamponade?

➢ Distant heart sounds, elevated jugular pressure, and hypotension

247. What is pulsus paradoxus? In which cardiac pathology is it associated with?

➢ An exaggerated fall in blood pressure during inspiration by >10 mmHg

➢ Pericardial tamponade

Metabolic & Endocrine

248. What is the classically described odor of a patient's breath with DKA? What ketone causes this?

➢ Sweet and fruity

➢ Acetone

249. Acanthosis nigricans is an indicator of what metabolic disorder?

➢ Insulin resistance

250. What is a common dermatologic finding manifesting around the eyes associated with hyperlipidemia?

➢ Xanthelasma palpabrum

251. What is the physical exam finding which causes thickening of tendons in patients with hyperlipidemia?

➢ Tendinous xanthomas

252. What is the Chvostek's signs? What may it suggest?
> Tapping of the facial nerve causes contraction of ipsilateral facial muscles
> May suggests of hypocalcemia

253. What is the Trousseau's sign? What may it suggest?
> Inflation of a blood pressure cuff above systolic blood pressure for 3 minutes leading to carpal spasm
> May suggests of hypocalcemia

Urogenital

254. What is a positive Prehn's sign? What does it suggest?
> Relief of testicular pain with elevation of the affected hemiscrotum
> Suggestive of epididymitis

Hip Pain

255. What are common risk factors for avascular necrosis of the hip?
> Alcohol use, glucocorticoid intra-articular administration, sickle cell disease, chronic renal failure, systemic lupus erythematosus, trauma

256. What are the common presenting signs and symptoms of femoral head pathologies and hip pain?
> Groin pain, buttock pain, thigh pain, and trouble ambulating

257. What is the initial diagnostic modality of choice for a patient with hip pain?
> Plain films of the hips
  ▪ Plain radiographs could remain normal months after symptoms, additional imaging with CT or MRI scans are warranted if symptoms persist

258. What is Noble's compression test?
> A provocative test to test for iliotibial band syndrome

259. What is the utility of the flexion adduction internal rotation (FADIR) test? Of a flexion abduction and external rotation (FABER) test?
> FADIR: Aid in diagnosis anterior hip impingement
> FABER: Aid in the diagnosis of osteoarthritis

Carpal Tunnel Syndrome

260. What is the hallmark presentation of carpal tunnel syndrome (CTS)?
> Numbness and tingling over the median nerve distribution (first 3 digits and radial side of the 4th)

261. What are the risk factors for carpal tunnel syndrome?
> Female gender, obesity, hypothyroidism, pregnancy, trauma, diabetes

262. How do you diagnose CTS?
> It is a clinical diagnosis and CTS is suspected when paresthesias are present in the median nerve distribution

263. What two modalities can be used to help diagnose CTS?
   - ➤ Provocative maneuvers: Phalen's and Tinel's test
   - ➤ Nerve conduction studies: Helps to identify patients with severe neuropathy

264. What are the treatment options for CTS?
   - ➤ Trial of nonsurgical treatment options first: Nocturnal wrist splinting and/or intra-articular glucocorticoid injections
   - ➤ Surgical decompression

265. What are the indications for surgical decompression of CTS?
   - ➤ Active denervation on nerve conduction studies, muscle weakness of thenar hypertrophy, or failure of nonsurgical treatment

Gout & Pseudogout

266. List the risk factors for developing gout?
   - ➤ Obesity, metabolic syndrome/insulin resistance, diabetes
   - ➤ Certain medications (ie. thiazide diuretics)
   - ➤ Alcohol in dose dependent manner
   - ➤ High purine diet (ie. red meat, shellfish seafood)

267. What are the three most common classes of medications used to treat gout flare?
   - ➤ NSAIDs, steroids, colchicine

268. What is the target serum urate level for patients with and without tophaceous gout?
   - ➤ <5 mg/dL with tophaceous gout
   - ➤ <6 mg/dL without tophaceous gout

269. What are the classic features of gout crystals seen on light microscopy?
    ➤ Negatively birefringent needle-shaped crystals
270. What are the classic features of calcium pyrophosphate crystal deposition (CPPD) pseudogout crystals seen on light microscopy?
    ➤ Positively birefringent rhomboid or rectangular crystals
271. What is the most common joint affected in CPPD?
    ➤ Knee
272. In the analysis of synovial fluid, what white count value differentiates a non-inflammatory versus a septic/inflammatory etiology?
    ➤ WBC >2000/mm³ suggest inflammatory or septic etiology

Knee Pain

273. What are common causes of anterior knee pain?
    ➤ Patellar subluxation or dislocation, tibial apophysitis, patellofemoral pain syndrome, patellar tendinitis
274. What are common causes of medial knee pain?
    ➤ Medial collateral ligament sprain, pes anserine bursitis, medial meniscus tear
275. What are common causes of lateral knee pain?
    ➤ Iliotibial band tendonitis, lateral meniscus tear, lateral collateral ligament tear
276. What are common causes of posterior knee pain?

> Popliteal cyst (Bakers cyst), posterior cruciate ligament tear

277. What is the classic presentation of a popliteal cyst (Bakers cyst)?

> Medial popliteal mass most prominent on standing or with knee fully flexed which can be painful or non-painful

278. What can severe symptoms of popliteal cyst mimic?

> Severe symptoms or ruptured cysts can mimic thrombophlebitis or DVT (ie. calf pain, swelling and warmth)

279. What is the first line treatment for an asymptomatic popliteal cyst? For a symptomatic popliteal cyst?

> Asymptomatic: No treatment required but provide education of small risk of future cyst rupture and if symptomatic then seek further medical evaluation

> Symptomatic: Conservative management (ie. treatment of underlying joint disorder such as osteoarthritis)

- If persistent symptoms, arthrocentesis of the knee and intraarticular injection with glucocorticoid

280. What physical exam can help in the diagnosis of a posterior cruciate ligament tear?

> Posterior drawer test

281. What physical exam can help in the diagnosis of anterior cruciate ligament tear?

> ➤ Anterior drawer, Lachman's, and Pivot shift tests

Reactive Arthritis

282. What is the triad of clinical symptoms often seen in reactive arthritis?
> ➤ Inflammatory arthritis of large joints
> ➤ Inflammation of the eyes (ie. conjunctivitis, uveitis)
> ➤ Inflammation of the GU tract (ie. urethritis, cervicitis)

283. What are four major musculoskeletal manifestations of reactive arthritis?
> ➤ Back pain, enthesitis, dactylitis, and arthritis

Miscellaneous

284. What are the signs and symptoms of lateral femoral cutaneous nerve entrapment syndrome (meralgia paresthetica)?
> ➤ Pain and paresthesia on the anterolateral thigh

285. What are the risk factors for lateral femoral cutaneous nerve entrapment syndrome? What are the treatment options?
> ➤ Diabetes, obesity, clothes with tight-fitting waist bands, pregnancy
> ➤ Encourage weight loss and looser fitting clothes

286. What is the hallmark presentation of Morton's neuroma?
> ➤ Burning pain in the inter-metatarsal space between the 3rd and 4th metatarsal that radiates towards the toes

287. What are the typical signs and symptoms of iliotibial band syndrome?

> Lateral knee pain worsened with climbing stairs or going uphill
> Tenderness over the lateral femoral condyle

288. Name the 4 muscles that make up the rotator cuff anatomy

> **S**upraspinatus, **I**nfraspinatus, **T**eres minor, **S**ubscapularis (**SITS**)

289. What are common symptoms and signs of plantar fasciitis?

> Pain in the inferior heel worsened with "first step" and point tenderness in that area on exam

290. What are the red flags for a vertebral fracture in a patient presenting with acute back pain?

> Contusions, older age, prolonged corticosteroid use, severe trauma, point tenderness

291. What are the classic physical exam findings on the hands in patients with nodal osteoarthritis?

> Heberden's (DIPJ) and Bouchard nodes (PIPJ)

Preoperative Evaluation for Noncardiac Surgery

292. What are considered low risk (<1%) surgical procedures?

> Cataract, dental, breast, superficial skin, minor urologic (TURP, TURBT), endoscopic, reconstructive/cosmetic, minor orthopedic, minor gynecologic, thyroid

293. What are considered high risk (>5%) surgical procedures?

> Lung, pancreas, liver transplantation, major vascular surgery, major abdominal surgery, esophagectomy, pneumonectomy, adrenal resection

294. What is the suggested timeframe for smoking cessation prior to surgery to reduce perioperative pulmonary complications?

> At least 4 weeks (preferably >8 weeks)

295. What perioperative comorbidities are associated with alcohol consumption?

> General infections, wound infections, pulmonary complications

296. What are the indications for obtaining preoperative platelet count?

> History of liver disease, bleeding diathesis, myeloproliferative disorders

297. What are the indications for obtaining preoperative coagulation labs such as prothrombin time (PT), partial thromboplastin (PTT), international normalized ratio (INR)?

> Malnutrition, warfarin use, heparin use, history of bleeding diathesis, liver disease, long-term antibiotic use

298. What are the indications for obtaining preoperative creatinine and blood urea nitrogen?

> Cardiac disease, major surgery, chronic kidney disease, hypertension, diabetes, medications that may affect renal function (ie. ACEi/ARB)

299. Name one indication for obtaining a preoperative liver function test?

> Cirrhosis

300. What are the indications for obtaining a preoperative electrocardiogram?

> Uncontrolled hypertension, known coronary artery disease, chronic kidney disease

301. What is an indication for obtaining a preoperative chest radiograph?

> Symptoms or exam findings suggestive of active cardiopulmonary disease

302. What are the indications for obtaining preoperative electrolytes?

> Congestive heart failure, known kidney disease, medications that can affect electrolytes (ie. diuretics)

303. What are the indications for obtaining a preoperative hemoglobin?

> Anticipation of major blood loss or symptoms of anemia

304. List some examples of validated preoperative risk assessment calculator tools?

> Revised Cardiac Risk Index (RCRI) calculator (well validated)

> American College of Surgeons National Surgical Quality Improvement Program (NSQIP) surgical risk calculator

> Myocardial infarction or cardiac arrest tool

305. What patient population is at risk for postoperative adrenal insufficiency and hypotension? How do you manage these patients perioperatively?

> Patient's taking the equivalent of >5 mg of prednisone daily for over 3 weeks within 6-12 months prior to surgery
> These patients should undergo cosyntropin stimulation testing prior to surgery
  - If positive results, recommend large stress-dose hydrocortisone at higher-than-physiologic doses with assistance of endocrinology specialty

306. What is the recommended perioperative management of beta blockers?

> Continue beta blockers if already on
> If starting, preferable to start >1 day ahead of surgery and titrate to effect (do not start on day of surgery)

307. What is the recommended perioperative management of alpha-2 agonist?

> Continue alpha-2 agonist if already on
> Do not start alpha-2 agonist if not already taking

308. What is the recommended perioperative management of calcium channel blockers?

> Continue calcium channel blockers if already on

309. What is the recommended perioperative management of ACEi/ARB?

> Hold on the morning of surgery
  - If the patient has heart failure, consider continuation of ACEi/ARB

310. What is the recommended perioperative management of glucocorticoids?

> Continue glucocorticoids if already on

311. What is the recommended perioperative management of aspirin?

> Safe to continue for dental or dermatologic procedures

> For more invasive procedures and if ASA is used for secondary prevention, a discussion about risk and benefits would be warranted with patient, cardiologist, and/or neurologist

312. What is the recommended perioperative management of coumadin in low-risk procedures?

> Hold 5 days prior to procedure

> Monitor INR

313. When should you restart coumadin after a procedure?

> 12-24 hours after surgery (typically the evening post-procedure if hemostasis has been achieved)

314. What is the recommended management of direct oral anticoagulants (DOACs) in patient's undergoing low, moderate or high-risk procedures?

> Hold 48 hours prior to high bleeding risk procedures

> Hold 24 hours prior to low or moderate risk bleeding procedures

315. When should you restart DOACs after a procedure?

> Restart 48 hours after high bleeding risk procedures

> ➤ Restart 24 hours after low or moderate risk
> bleeding procedures

2

CARDIOLOGY

General Cardiology

316. What are the common causes of pericardial tamponade?
> ➤ Idiopathic, malignancy, uremia, aortic dissection, myocardial wall rupture

317. What are the common causes of pericarditis?
> ➤ Malignancy, uremia, idiopathic, TB, bacterial, viral, post-surgical

318. What are the risk factors for acute aortic dissections?
> ➤ HTN, male sex, cocaine use, connective tissue disease (ie. Marfan's), aortitis (ie. Takayasu, syphilis, giant cell arteritis), trauma

319. What is first line medical therapy for acute aortic dissection?
> ➤ IV beta blockers

Coronary Artery Disease & Electrocardiogram Abnormalities

320. What study is the gold standard to evaluate obstructive coronary artery disease?
> ➤ Coronary angiography

321. What is the definition of stable angina?
> ➤ Substernal chest pain or discomfort aggravated by exercise and alleviated by rest or administration of nitroglycerin

322. What is the definition of unstable angina?
> ➤ Acute chest pain or discomfort while at rest

323. What are two methods of performing cardiac stress testing?

> Exercise or pharmacologic

324. What are the indications for pharmacologic stress testing rather than exercise stress testing?

> Patients that are unable to walk on the treadmill, recent myocardial infarction, presence of a left bundle branch block

325. What are contraindications to cardiac stress testing?

> Acute myocardial infarction within the past 48 hours, acute pulmonary embolism, unstable angina, severe symptomatic aortic stenosis, uncontrolled heart failure and arrhythmias

326. What are classic findings of a RBBB on ECG?

> QRS ≥120 msec, RSR' in V1-V3, wide/slurred S wave in lateral leads (I, aVL, V5, and V6)

327. What are the most common etiologies of left ventricular hypertrophy?

> Hypertension, aortic stenosis/insufficiency, coarctation of the aorta, hypertrophic cardiomyopathy

328. What are the most common etiologies of right ventricular hypertrophy?

> Mitral valve stenosis, tricuspid regurgitation, pulmonary hypertension, congenital (ie. tetralogy of Fallot, ventricular septal defect, transposition of the great arteries)

329. What are the ECG criteria for ST elevation myocardial infarction?

> New ST-elevation at the J-point in 2 contiguous leads with the cut-point ≥1 mm in all leads other than leads V2–V3 where the following cut-points apply:
  - ≥2 mm in men ≥40 years
  - ≥2.5 mm in men <40 years
  - ≥1.5 mm in women regardless of age

330. What are contraindications to fibrinolysis?

> History of intracranial hemorrhage, neoplasms, aneurysm, non-hemorrhagic stroke or closed head trauma within 3 months, active bleeding or known bleeding diathesis

331. What are the most common mechanical complications following a myocardial infarction?

> Ventricular septal defect, left ventricle free wall rupture, papillary muscle rupture

332. What is the most common distribution of a myocardial infarction that leads to papillary muscle rupture?

> Inferior myocardial infarction

333. What are the signs and symptoms of Dressler's syndrome?

> 2-10 weeks post-MI with pleuritis, fever, and pericarditis

334. What are the common etiologies of dilated cardiomyopathy?

> Valvular disease, toxic (ie. alcohol, cocaine, trastuzumab), infiltrative, stress induced, metabolic (ie. hypothyroidism)

335. What is a common auscultatory murmur in hypertrophic cardiomyopathy?

> Increased systolic murmur along left lower sternal border with Valsalva and standing

336. What coronary artery is commonly affected in a septal wall myocardial infarction?

> Proximal left anterior descending

337. What ECG leads show ST elevation changes in septal wall myocardial infarction?

> V1 and V2

338. What coronary artery is commonly affected in an anterior wall myocardial infarction?

> Left anterior descending

339. What ECG leads show ST elevation changes in an anterior wall myocardial infarction?

> V3 and V4

340. What coronary artery is commonly affected in an apical wall myocardial infarction?

> Distal left anterior descending

341. What coronary artery is commonly affected in lateral wall myocardial infarction?

> Left circumflex

342. What ECG leads show ST elevation changes in lateral wall myocardial infarction?

> I and aVL, V5, and V6

343. What coronary artery is commonly affected in an inferior wall myocardial infarction?

> Right coronary artery in most patients
>   - In a left dominant coronary circulation, it can occur due to the left circumflex artery

344. What ECG leads show ST elevation changes in an inferior wall myocardial infarction?

> II, III, and aVF

345. What coronary artery is commonly affected in a right ventricular wall myocardial infarction?

> Proximal right coronary artery (proximal to the RV marginal branch)

346. What ECG leads show ST elevation changes in right ventricular wall myocardial infarction?

> V1, V2, and a reversed V4 lead

347. What coronary artery is commonly affected in a posterior myocardial infarction?

> Right coronary or left circumflex depending on dominance (whichever artery the posterior descending artery arises from)

348. What ECG leads show ST elevation changes in a posterior myocardial infarction?

> V1-V3

349. What is Prinzmetal angina?

> Coronary artery vasospasm with transient ST elevation

350. What are the first-line treatments for Prinzmetal angina (coronary vasospasm)?

> Calcium channel blockers and nitrates

351. What is the time goal for reperfusion in a patient with ACS?

> PCI within 90 minutes of first contact

352. In a non-PCI capable hospital that is >120 minutes away from the closest PCI center, what

therapy should be administered for management of ST elevation myocardial infarction?

> Fibrinolytic

353. What medications are indicated for post myocardial infarction?

> Beta blockers, aspirin, P2Y12 inhibitor, high intensity statin, ACE inhibitor

Arrhythmias

354. What are the common metabolic disorders that can cause sinus bradycardia?

> Sepsis, hypothermia, hypoxia, and hypoglycemia

355. What ECG findings are seen in 1st, 2nd, and 3rd degree heart blocks?

> 1st degree: PR interval prolongation >200 ms
> 2nd degree:
  - Type 1 (Mobitz I/Wenckebach): Progressively increasing PR interval leading to dropped QRS complex
    • Remember: "Dance, do the Wenckebach - longer, longer, longer, drop"
  - Type 2 (Mobitz II): Constant PR interval with random dropped QRS complexes
> 3rd degree: Absence of AV conduction

356. What is the anatomical location of the primary pathology in Mobitz I?

> AV node abnormality

357. What is the anatomical location of the primary pathology in Mobitz II?

> His-Purkinje abnormality

358. What is the classic ECG finding of a 3rd degree heart block?

  ➢ AV dissociation

359. What are common types of supraventricular tachycardias (SVTs)?

  ➢ Atrial fibrillation, atrial flutter, multifocal atrial tachycardia, AV nodal reentry tachycardia, AV reentrant tachycardia

360. What change to the QRS complex occurs with SVT? When might this not be true?

  ➢ Narrow complex QRS
  ➢ Preexcitation or aberrancy, which then may widen the QRS complex

361. What classic pulmonary disease is associated with multifocal atrial tachycardia?

  ➢ COPD

362. What is the first line treatment for an unstable patient with SVT?

  ➢ Cardioversion

363. How do you define an accessory pathway?

  ➢ An abnormal pathway of conduction between two parts of the heart

364. What is the abnormality found in Wolff-Parkinson-White Syndrome?

  ➢ Bundle of Kent accessory pathway which connects the atria to the ventricles

365. What are classic ECG findings of the Wolff-Parkinson-White accessory pathway?

> PR interval <120 ms (short PR interval), slurring
> of the onset of the QRS (delta wave), and
> increased QRS duration due to slurred upstroke

366. What are two common etiologies of wide complex
tachycardias?

> Ventricular tachycardia
> SVT with aberrant conduction

367. What are the two types of ventricular tachycardia?

> Monomorphic
> Polymorphic

Atrial Fibrillation (AF)

368. What is the most common clinically significant
arrhythmia?

> Atrial fibrillation (AF)

369. How is AF classified?

> Paroxysmal: AF which terminates spontaneously
> or with intervention within 7 days of onset
> Persistent: Continuous AF that is sustained >7
> days
> Long-standing persistent: Continuous AF >12
> months
> Permanent: When the clinician and patient
> mutually decide that rhythm control will not be
> further attempted and the patient will remain in
> atrial fibrillation

370. Is AF more prevalent in men or women?

> Men

371. What are the common presenting symptoms of
AF?

> Chest pain, palpitations, shortness of breath, and fatigue

372. What are the pathognomonic ECG changes seen in AF?

> Absence of P waves and the presence of an "irregularly irregular rhythm"
  - Ventricular rhythm with no specific pattern

373. What hormone level should always be checked in a patient with newly diagnosed AF?

> Thyroid-stimulating hormone (TSH)

374. What is the role of obtaining a transthoracic echocardiogram in newly diagnosed AF?

> Identify underlying structural heart disease, left atrial appendage thrombus, and to evaluate for tachycardia induced cardiomyopathy

375. What intervention should be considered in a hemodynamically **stable** patient with AF with rapid ventricular response? Hemodynamically unstable patient?

> Rate control with beta blockers or calcium channel blockers

376. What intervention should be considered in a hemodynamically **unstable** patient with AF with rapid ventricular response?

> Synchronized cardioversion

377. What are the two primary cardiovascular complications of AF?

> Cardiomyopathy and thromboembolism

378. What is the most common arterial thromboembolic complication of AF?

> Stroke

379. What was the outcome of the AFFIRM trial with regards to mortality?

> All-cause mortality was equal in the rate and rhythm control cohorts

380. What is the resting heart rate goal in the treatment of AF? What trial was this based on?

> ≤110 beats/minute
> RACE2

381. What are the first line therapies for rate control in AF?

> Beta blockers and non-dihydropyridine calcium channel blockers
  - Newer data suggests rhythm control with DCCV + ablation may be better

382. What are the preferred non-dihydropyridine calcium channel blockers for rate control in AF?

> Diltiazem and verapamil

383. What should be evaluated for prior to elective direct current or pharmacologic cardioversion?

> Presence of an atrial thrombus

384. What are the contraindications in the use of flecainide and propafenone?

> Structural heart disease

385. What are the side effects of amiodarone?

> Bradycardia, QT prolongation, pulmonary toxicity, and hyperthyroidism

386. Where does arrhythmogenic activity most commonly originate in the development of AF?

> Pulmonary veins

387. What risk does the CHA_2DS_2VASc score calculate?

> ➤ Yearly stroke risk in a patient with AF

388. What are the components of the CHA_2DS_2VASc score?

> ➤ **C**ongestive heart failure (1pt)
> ➤ **H**ypertension (1pt)
> ➤ **A**ge ≥75 years (**2pts**)
> ➤ **D**iabetes mellitus (1pt)
> ➤ **S**troke/TIA (history of) (**2pts**)
> ➤ **V**ascular disease (1pt)
> ➤ **A**ge 65-74 (1pt)
> ➤ **S**ex **c**ategory (female) (1pt)

389. At what CHA_2DS_2VASc score is anticoagulation definitely indicated?

> ➤ ≥2

390. What are common drugs that can precipitate AF?

> ➤ Cocaine, amphetamines, caffeine, theophylline

391. What are common pulmonary comorbidities that can precipitate AF?

> ➤ COPD, pulmonary embolism, obstructive sleep apnea, hypoxia

392. What are the non-drug therapies for the management of AF? For more refractory cases?

> ➤ Catheter ablation of the pulmonary veins (pulmonary vein isolation) or any other focus of abnormal electrical activity
> ➤ Refractory cases: Permanent pacemaker insertion and catheter ablation of the AV node can be performed

393. What are the major complications of catheter ablation?

> Cardiac perforation, pulmonary vein stenosis, atrioesophageal fistula, and stroke

394. What is the drug of choice in patients with AF and valvular disease (ie. severe mitral stenosis, mechanical prosthetic valve)?

> Warfarin (coumadin)

395. What are the drugs of choice in patients with AF without valvular disease (non-valvular AF)?

> Direct-Acting Oral Anticoagulants (DOAC): Apixaban, rivaroxaban, dabigatran, edoxaban

396. What is the method of choice to decrease stroke risk in a patient who cannot tolerate blood thinners?

> Occlusion of the left atrial appendage

Heart Failure (HF)

397. What are the three subclassifications of heart failure according to left ventricular ejection fraction (LVEF)?

> Heart failure with preserved ejection fraction (HFpEF): LVEF ≥50%
> Heart failure with midrange ejection fraction (HFmrEF): LVEF 41%-49%
> Heart failure reduced ejection fraction (HFrEF): LVEF ≤40%

398. How is severity of heart failure symptoms graded and what are the subclassifications?

> New York Heart Association (NYHA) functional class designation

- Class I: No limitation in normal physical activity
- Class II: Mild symptoms only during normal activity
- Class III: Marked symptoms during daily activity, comfortable at rest
- Class IV: Severe limitations and symptoms even at rest

399. What initial testing should be obtained if the diagnosis of HFrEF fraction is suspected? What test is used to confirm the diagnosis?

➤ Chest x-ray, electrocardiogram, natriuretic peptides

➤ Transthoracic echocardiogram (TTE)

400. What is the most common cause of HFrEF?

➤ Ischemia

401. What radiographic signs are suggestive of HFrEF on chest x-ray?

➤ Bilateral pleural effusions, pulmonary edema (ie. peribronchial cuffing, Kerley B lines, alveolar edema), enlarged cardiac silhouette

402. What five classes of medication have shown to reduce morbidity and mortality in HFrEF?

➤ Angiotensin-converting enzyme inhibitors (ACEi)

➤ Angiotensin II receptor blockers (ARB)

➤ Angiotensin receptor-Neprilysin inhibitor (ARNI)

➤ Beta blockers

➤ Mineralocorticoid receptor antagonist (MRA)

403. Which beta blockers have been shown to reduce mortality in HF?

> Metoprolol succinate, carvedilol, and bisoprolol

404. What two MRA are used in the treatment of HFrEF?

> Spironolactone and eplerenone

405. When are the indications to initiate MRA in a patient with HFrEF?

> In conjunction with an ACEi/ARB, or ARNI, and beta blocker in patients with a LVEF <35% and NYHA class II-IV symptoms

406. What are contraindications in starting MRA in patients with HFrEF?

> Baseline serum creatinine level >2.5 mg/dL (or eGFT <30 mL/min/1.73m²) or serum potassium >5.0 meq/L

407. What medication reduces all-cause mortality in African American patients with persistent symptomatic heart failure with LVEF ≤35%? What study supports this?

> Hydralazine/isosorbide dinitrate
> African American Heart Failure Trial (A-HeFT)

408. What are the indications for cardiac resynchronization therapy?

> LVEF <35%, normal sinus rhythm with a QRS duration of >150 ms and a LBBB, and NYHA Class II or greater

409. What exam findings are specific for HFrEF?

> Elevated jugular venous pressure, positive abdominojugular reflux (increase in JVP of >3

cm, sustained for >15 seconds), audible S3 (ventricular gallop), laterally displaced apical impulse

410. What are the most typical signs and symptoms of HFrEF?

> Dyspnea, reduced exercise tolerance, fatigue, paroxysmal nocturnal dyspnea, orthopnea, and ankle swelling

411. Which class of anti-diabetic medications has been shown to decrease all cause and cardiovascular mortality?

> SGLT-2 inhibitors

412. What are the two most commonly used SGLT-2 inhibitors prescribed in the US?

> Dapagliflozin and empagliflozin

413. What is the preferred class of diuretics in management of patients with chronic HFrEF?

> Loop diuretics

414. What are the two natriuretic peptide biomarkers used in heart failure?

> B-type natriuretic peptide (BNP) and its precursor N-terminal pro-B-type natriuretic peptide (NT-proBNP)

415. What value of NT-proBNP and BNP may rule **out** acute heart failure?

> NT-proBNP <300 pg/mL, BNP <100 pg/mL

416. What value of NT-proBNP and BNP may rule **in** acute heart failure?

> NT-proBNP >450 pg/mL (patient <50 years)

> NT-proBNP >900 pg/mL (patient 50-75 years)

> NT-proBNP >1800 pg/mL (>75 years)

> BNP >500 pg/mL

417. What factors can artificially decrease natriuretic peptides?

> Obesity, pericardial constriction, and the use of ARNI medications (Sacubitril-Valsartan)

418. What factors (other than HF) increase natriuretic peptides?

> Advancing age, atrial fibrillation and other arrhythmias, and kidney failure

419. What is the mechanism of action of Ivabradine?

> Inhibits pacemaker activity in the sinoatrial node by blocking the funny channel (Na-K) current

420. What are the contraindications to starting ivabradine?

> Decompensated HF, BP <90/50 mmHg, conduction abnormality, HR <60

421. Which medication class has been shown generate the highest mortality reduction in HFrEF?

> ARNI

422. What is the duration and why is there a washout period between transitioning from an ACEi to an ARNI?

> 36 hours to prevent angioedema

423. How quickly should beta blockers be up-titrated in stable patients?

> Every 1-2 weeks

424. When should a TTE be repeated in a patient with HFrEF?

➢ After 3-6 months of guideline directed medical therapy

Valvular Heart Disease

425. What are the common etiologies of aortic stenosis in older patients? Younger patients?

➢ Older patients: Age related calcifications

➢ Younger patients: Bicuspid aortic valve

426. What are the common etiologies of mitral valve stenosis?

➢ Mitral annular calcifications, rheumatic heart disease, congenital, infectious endocarditis (large lesions), lupus, amyloid

427. In rheumatic heart disease, the mitral valve is often described as having what appearance?

➢ Fish mouth

428. What are the common etiologies of aortic insufficiency?

➢ Bicuspid aortic valve, infective endocarditis, aortic root disease, rheumatic heart disease

429. What are common etiologies of mitral valve prolapse?

➢ Connective tissue diseases (ie. Ehlers-Danlos and Marfan's), familial, and idiopathic

430. What are the common etiologies of tricuspid valve regurgitation?

➢ Connective tissue diseases, infective endocarditis, Ebstein's anomaly, rheumatic heart disease

431. What are the two types of prosthetic heart valves?

> Bioprosthetic
> Mechanical

432. What are the two types of bioprosthetic heart valves?

> Bovine
> Porcine

433. What is the difference in durability of bioprosthetic and mechanical heart valves?

> Mechanical: Very durable, typically 20-30 year lifespan
> Bioprosthetic: Less durable, typically 10 year lifespan

434. Which prosthetic heart valve requires anticoagulation?

> Mechanical

435. What anticoagulant is currently the first line therapy for patients with a mechanical aortic valve?

> Coumadin

436. What is the INR goal in a patient with a mechanical aortic valve with no heart failure or AF?

> 2.0-3.0

437. What is the INR goal in a patient with a mechanical aortic valve with atrial fibrillation or chronic heart failure?

> 2.5-3.5

438. What is the INR goal in a patient with a mechanical mitral valve?

> 2.5-3.5

Infective Endocarditis

439. What imaging test is indicated if you suspect infective endocarditis and the transthoracic echocardiogram is negative or non-diagnostic?

> Transesophageal echocardiogram

440. What cardiac conditions predispose a person to infective endocarditis?

> Rheumatic heart disease
> - Most common cause in developing countries
> Prosthetic valves and degenerative valve disease (mitral regurgitation associated with degenerative mitral valve prolapse is the most common in developed countries), bicuspid aortic valve, aortic stenosis, and ventricular septal defects

441. What are the two classic features of infective endocarditis?

> Fever and heart murmur
> - Each found in >80% of patients

442. What are the typical causative microorganisms in native valve infective endocarditis?

> Gram-positive bacteria (80% of cases)
> Staphylococcus aureus, streptococcus gallolyticus, streptococcus viridans, and HACEK organisms (haemophilus species, aggregatibacter species, cardiobacterium species, eikenella corrodens, kingella species)

443. What are the components of the Modified Duke Criteria for the clinical diagnosis of infective endocarditis?

> Major criteria:

- Positive blood cultures from typical organisms
  - 2 separate cultures drawn >12 hrs apart **OR**
  - At least 3 of ≥4 blood cultures taken at least 1 hr apart **OR**
  - A single positive culture for coxiella burnetii
- Echocardiographic findings positive for IE (ie. vegetations)

➢ Minor criteria: Predisposing cardiac condition, fever, vascular or immunologic phenomenon on physical exam, positive blood cultures that do not meet major criteria

444. What is the antibiotic treatment of choice for native-valve infective endocarditis caused by methicillin-susceptible Staphylococcus aureus?

➢ Beta lactams (ie. oxacillin or nafcillin)

445. What are the most common causes of blood culture negative infective endocarditis?

➢ Recent administration of antibiotics

➢ Fastidious or hard to culture infectious organisms (ie. HACEK organisms or fungal infections)

➢ Poor microbiologic technique upon collection and culture

446. What is the treatment of choice for native-valve infective endocarditis due to methicillin resistant staphylococcus aureus (MRSA)?

➢ Monotherapy with daptomycin or vancomycin

447. What are the three main indications for surgery in native valve endocarditis?

> Heart failure due to valvular dysfunction,
uncontrolled infection, and prevention of
systemic embolization especially in the setting of
a large vegetation (>10 mm)

448. What is the treatment of choice for enterococcal
infective endocarditis?

> Combination therapy with penicillin or
ampicillin with gentamicin
  - In elderly patients consider ampicillin and
  ceftriaxone due to gentamicin toxicity

3

CRITICAL CARE

ICU 101

449. What are the two main benefits of an arterial line?
    ➤ Closer hemodynamic monitoring of blood pressure
    ➤ Frequent ABGs for patients on ventilator

450. What are the main benefits of noninvasive positive pressure ventilation (BIPAP) as compared to non-rebreather facemask?
    ➤ Improves ventilation and gas exchange in patients with hypercarbic respiratory failure
    ➤ Decreases preload and afterload

451. What are contraindications to noninvasive positive pressure ventilation?
    ➤ Vomiting
    ➤ Inability to protect airway
    ➤ Agitated patient
    ➤ Facial trauma

452. What type of IV access should be obtained in a patient that is admitted to the medical ICU for hemorrhagic shock from a variceal bleed?
    ➤ Two peripheral 16-gauge IVs or central venous access with an introducer catheter for rapid blood infusion

453. What additional causes of hypoxia for a ventilated patient should be considered?
    ➤ **D**isplacement of ET Tube
    ➤ **O**bstruction (ie. mucus plug)
    ➤ **P**neumothorax
    ➤ **E**quipment malfunction

> **S**tacking breaths ("auto-PEEP")
  - Remember: "**DOPES**"

454. What is air stacking (or auto-PEEP)?
  > When a mechanically ventilated patient does not exhale completely before initiating their next breath, which leads to air trapping, and an increase in alveolar pressure at end of expiration

455. What are potential sequelae of air stacking?
  > Decreased venous return, cardiac output, and hypotension
  > Alveolar overdistension and increased barotrauma and ventilator associated lung injury

456. What may be observed on the ventilator when auto-PEEP is occurring?
  > Continuous expiratory flow all the way until the start of inspiration

457. What parameters can be changed on the ventilator to reduce auto-PEEP?
  > Reduce respiratory rate
  > Reduce tidal volume
  > Increase inspiratory flow rate
  > Increase expiratory time

458. Why is hydrocortisone used for stress dose steroids? What is the dose?
  > It has both glucocorticoid and mineralocorticoid activity
  > 50 mg q6h

459. To minimize the length of time patients remain intubated, what two things should be done every day in the ICU (unless there is a contraindication)?

> Sedation holiday
> Spontaneous breathing trial

460. What are five ways to confirm correct endotracheal tube placement (ETT)?

> Bilateral breath sounds with symmetric chest rise
> Capnography
> Condensation in the endotracheal tube
> Chest x-ray
> Direct visualization with bronchoscopy

461. On a ventilator, what two basic parameters are responsible for oxygenation?

> FiO_2
> PEEP

462. On a ventilator, what two basic parameters are responsible for ventilation (ie. CO_2 exchange)?

> Respiratory rate
> Tidal volume or inspiratory pressure (depending on ventilator settings)

463. What is a plateau pressure?

> It is the pressure present in small airways and alveoli
  ▪ It is an estimate of lung compliance

464. How is a plateau pressure obtained?

> Apply an inspiratory breath hold on the ventilator, resulting in no flow and allowing the pressure measured by the ventilator to be equal to the pressure in the small airways

465. If the peak pressure is elevated, but the plateau pressure is normal, where is the pathology located?

> In the airways

466. What are examples of pathologies that result in elevated peak pressures with normal plateau pressures?

> Bronchospasm
> Mucus plugs/secretions
> Kinked ETT
> Patient biting tube

467. What are examples of pathologies that result in elevated plateau pressures?

> ARDS
> Pneumonia
> Pneumothorax
> Pulmonary edema
> Atelectasis

468. What are adverse effects of tidal volumes that are too high?

> Barotrauma
> Respiratory alkalosis
> Decreased cardiac output

469. What medication, route of delivery, and dose should be administered to a patient who presents with anaphylaxis after a bee sting.?

> Intramuscular epinephrine, 1:1000 preparation, 0.3-0.5 mg

470. What is abdominal compartment syndrome? How can it be assessed?

> Sustained intra-abdominal pressure >20 mmHg associated with new organ dysfunction

> Can be measured from bladder pressure via a
foley

471. What should be done next for a young person
who is an active intravenous drug user and
presents unresponsive and has improvement with
return to normal mental status with IV naloxone
bolus?

> Continue to observe the patient for several
hours as the half-life of naloxone is short, and
patient could become obtunded again after the
medication wears off

472. What is the goal glucose in ICU patients?

> ≤180 mg/dL

- Tight glucose control (glucose <108 mg/dL) in
ICU patients increases mortality (NICE-Sugar
trial)

473. How soon after admission should nutrition be
started for a patient who is admitted to the ICU
with septic shock? What route of feeding should
be used?

> Within 24-48 hours

> Enteral nutrition

474. In a critically ill patient who previously was well
nourished and cannot tolerate enteral feeding
(either due to ileus, mechanical obstruction, or
alternative issue), how soon does parenteral
nutrition need to be started?

> Not sooner than day 7 of an acute illness

475. What is one of the major adverse effects of total parental nutrition and a major reason why we do not rush to start it in critically ill patients?
    ➤ Increased risks for infections, specifically fungemia

476. What is the likely diagnosis for a previously healthy patient that was hospitalized for two weeks in the ICU with COVID-19 pneumonia and ARDS that is now extubated, awake, alert and on only 2L of oxygen via nasal cannula but remains extremely weak, not even able to lift themselves from laying to sitting without assistance?
    ➤ Critical illness myopathy

477. What causes malignant hyperthermia? What is the treatment?
    ➤ Allergic reaction to volatile anesthetic
    ➤ Treatment: Stop inciting drug, dantrolene

478. What are the five "can't miss" diagnoses for a patient presenting with acute onset chest pain?
    ➤ Myocardial infarction
    ➤ Pulmonary embolus
    ➤ Aortic dissection
    ➤ Pneumothorax
    ➤ Esophageal rupture

479. What is the treatment for a young patient who presents obtunded and is admitted to the ICU with suspected aspirin overdose?
    ➤ Urine alkalization
    ➤ Hemodialysis

480. If a patient has refractory alcohol withdrawal despite benzodiazepines, what medication can be used? If phenobarbital still is not reducing the patient's symptoms, what is the next step?
   ➤ Phenobarbital
   ➤ Intubate and start propofol drip
481. On lung ultrasound, what will be seen diffusely in all lung fields in a patient intubated for pulmonary edema?
   ➤ B-Lines

Cardiac Arrest & ACLS

482. How long is each cycle of CPR?
   ➤ Two minutes
483. Once the pads are placed on a patient, do you complete two full minutes of CPR before checking the rhythm or stop to analyze the rhythm immediately?
   ➤ Stop to analyze the rhythm immediately
484. What is the dose of epinephrine and how often is it given during CPR?
   ➤ 1 mg every 3-5 minutes
485. In a cardiac arrest, what two rhythms should be defibrillated?
   ➤ Ventricular fibrillation (VF)
   ➤ Pulseless ventricular tachycardia (VT)
486. When is amiodarone first given during a cardiac arrest? What is the dose?
   ➤ It is given in the third cycle of CPR (after epinephrine has been given) when there is refractory VT/VF

➤ 300 mg IV Push

487. In what scenario, according to ACLS protocol, should synchronized cardioversion be performed?

> ➤ Any patient with a pulse, that has unstable vitals (defined by hypotension, decreased consciousness, shock, or chest pain)

488. In ACLS protocol, what medications/interventions can be used for a patient with unstable bradycardia?

> ➤ **D**opamine
> ➤ **A**tropine
> ➤ **T**ranscutaneous pacing
> ➤ **E**pinephrine
>   ▪ Remember: "**DATE**"

Shock

489. What are the four main types of shock?

> ➤ Hemorrhagic
> ➤ Distributive (ie. septic, neurogenic, anaphylactic)
> ➤ Cardiogenic
> ➤ Obstructive

490. According to surviving sepsis guidelines, how much crystalloid fluid should be given for resuscitation in a patient with septic shock?

> ➤ 20-30 cc/kg crystalloid

491. What is the preferred vasopressor for treatment of septic shock?

> ➤ Norepinephrine

492. What is the mechanism of action for norepinephrine?

> Alpha 1 and beta 1 agonist (alpha 1 > beta 1)

493. What is mechanism of action for epinephrine?

> Alpha 1 and beta 1 agonist, beta 2 agonist (< alpha 1 and beta 1)

494. What is the mechanism of action for phenylephrine?

> Pure alpha 1 agonist

495. What is the mechanism of action for vasopressin?

> V1 and V2 receptor agonist

496. In cardiogenic shock, are the cardiac output (CO), preload, and systemic vascular resistance (SVR) high or low? In hypovolemic shock? In distributive shock?

> Cardiogenic shock:
  - **CO: Low – primary problem**
  - Preload: High
  - SVR: High
> Hypovolemic shock:
  - CO: Low
  - **Preload: Low – primary problem**
  - SVR: High
> Distributive shock:
  - CO: High
  - Preload: Low or normal
  - **SVR: Low – primary problem**

497. What physical exam finding can be a proxy of SVR?

> Physical extremities warmth (low SVR) vs cold (high SVR)

498. What physical exam finding can be a surrogate for preload?

➢ Juglar venous pressure

499. What physical exam finding can be a surrogate for cardiac output?

> ➢ High pulse pressure with bounding pulse: High cardiac output
> ➢ Low pulse pressure with thready pulse: Low cardiac output

500. If a patient is on the flat portion of the Frank-Starling curve, what does that suggest?

> ➢ No more fluids should be given, and vasopressors should be started if the patient remains hypotensive

Acute Respiratory Distress Syndrome (ARDS)

501. What is acute respiratory distress syndrome (ARDS)?

> ➢ Diffuse alveolar damage resulting from increased alveolar capillary permeability and non-cardiogenic pulmonary edema

502. What is the goal tidal volume for patients with ARDS according to ARDSnet protocol?

> ➢ 6-8 cc/kg of ideal body weight

503. What acid-base disturbance may need to be tolerated to adhere to goal tidal volumes for patients with ARDS?

> ➢ Permissive acidemia due to hypercarbia

504. What other intervention in ARDS has been shown to reduce mortality in some studies?

> Prone positioning

505. In severe ARDS, what is the PaO2/FiO2 ratio, when measured with a PEEP of 5?

> ≤100 mmHg

506. What is the goal plateau pressure in ARDS?

> <30 cm H_2O

507. If a patient with severe ARDS is going to be paralyzed to improve ventilator synchrony, what is essential to be done first?

> Deep sedation with BIS monitoring

Malignant Hypertension

508. What beta blocker should be used in acute aortic dissection?

> Esmolol

509. What is the definition of hypertensive emergency? What is the treatment (excluding aortic dissection, preeclampsia or pheochromocytoma crisis)?

> BP >180/120 with evidence of end-organ damage

> SBP reduced 25% in first hour, and if remains stable, reduce to 160/100 within 2-6 hours

510. Why should you avoid reducing the blood pressure too quickly in hypertensive emergency?

> It can cause ischemia in organs that have been habituated to higher levels of blood pressure

511. What is the blood pressure goal in a patient with hypertensive emergency and aortic dissection?

> SBP <120 mmHg within the first hour

- This is an exception to the above rule to reduce aortic shearing forces

512. Why should beta blockers be avoided in patients with cocaine use?
   ➢ It can precipitate unopposed alpha stimulation and lead to hypertensive emergency

513. In a patient with ACS and hypertensive emergency, what anti-hypertensive should be used as first line treatment?
   ➢ IV nitroglycerin

Venous Thromboembolism

514. What is Virchow's Triad?
   ➢ Stasis
   ➢ Hypercoagulability
   ➢ Endothelial damage

515. At what Wells score can a serum D-dimer be used to rule out pulmonary embolus (PE)?
   ➢ Wells score ≤4

516. What is the treatment for a non-massive pulmonary embolus?
   ➢ Anticoagulation

517. How is a massive pulmonary embolus defined? What is the treatment?
   ➢ PE with hypotension, cardiac arrest, or shock
   ➢ Treatment: Systemic tPA followed by heparin

518. When evaluating for a pulmonary embolus, how can an echocardiogram and biomarkers be helpful?

> If positive for right heart strain, they can assist in risk stratification and consideration of thrombolytic therapy

519. Why is it important to distinguish sub-massive PEs?

> These patients may benefit from thrombolytic therapy (either systemic or catheter directed)
>   - They often require a multidisciplinary approach between pulmonary, interventional radiology, and cardiothoracic surgery
> They also can be at higher risk for long-term sequelae such as chronic thromboembolic pulmonary hypertension (CTEPH)

Miscellaneous

520. What is the appropriate treatment for a patient that is found down next to a propane fueled heater and is nonresponsive with a pulse oximetry of 100%?

> Hyperbaric oxygen for carbon monoxide poisoning

521. Other than carbon monoxide, what can give you a falsely normal pulse oximetry reading?

> Cyanide poisoning

522. What is the treatment for cyanide poisoning?

> Hydroxocobalamin

523. What blood marker can be checked to exclude cyanide poisoning in a patient exposed to a fire?

> LDH (normal value excludes cyanide poisoning)

524. What are the classic signs and symptoms in hepatopulmonary syndrome?

➢ Platypnea

➢ Orthodeoxia

525. What is seen on echocardiogram with bubble study in patients with hepatopulmonary syndrome?

➢ Late bubbles passing into the left side of the heart after 4-5 cardiac cycles

526. What is the differential for an anterior mediastinal mass?

➢ **T**hymoma

➢ **T**horacic aorta aneurysm

➢ **T**eratoma/germ cell tumor

➢ **T**hyroid tissue (ectopic)

➢ **T**errible lymphoma

▪ Remember: "**Terrible T's**"

527. What medication should be administered when a patient is suspected of having high altitude cerebral edema?

➢ Dexamethasone

528. What medication can be used for high altitude pulmonary edema?

➢ Nifedipine

➢ Sildenafil

529. Following serial negative inspiratory force (a marker of inspiratory muscle strength) values over time can be helpful in what type of pulmonary disorders?

➢ Neuromuscular disorders

530. For a patient who has granulomatosis with polyangiitis who presents with diffuse alveolar hemorrhage, what would you expect their DLCO to be (decreased, normal, or increased)?

➤ Increased

531. What is the value of the 6-minute walk test?

➤ It can assess a patient's disability
➤ Can be used to determine need for supplemental oxygen
➤ Can be used to guide prognosis in patients with chronic lung disease
➤ Utilized as a standardized value for comparison in clinical trials

532. What are the common causes of a pleural fluid amylase level being greater than a serum amylase level?

➤ Pancreatic disease (ie. pancreatitis, cancer)
➤ Esophageal rupture

533. At what size is no follow up needed for a patient with no risk factors that is found to have a solitary pulmonary nodule?

➤ <6 mm

534. What is the first thing that should be done when assessing a pulmonary nodule that is found incidentally on a CT scan?

➤ Compare to prior scans

535. According to USPSTF guidelines, which patients should receive a low dose chest CT for lung cancer screening?

➤ Adults age 50-80 years
➤ 20 pack year smoking history
➤ Currently smoke, or have quit in the last 15 years

4

ENDOCRINOLOGY

Disorders of the Thyroid

General

536. What is the most sensitive test to detect primary hypo or hyperthyroidism?
   ➢ TSH

537. What comorbidities may lead to an increased thyroxine-binding globulin (TBG)?
   ➢ **H**epatitis
   ➢ **O**pioids
   ➢ **P**regnancy
   ➢ **E**strogens
      ▪ Remember: "**HOPE**"

538. What comorbidities may lead to a decrease in TBG?
   ➢ Nephritic syndrome
   ➢ Cirrhosis
   ➢ Androgens
   ➢ Glucocorticoids

539. What is the pattern of TSH, free T4, and T3 in sick euthyroid syndrome?
   ➢ All are decreased
   ➢ T3 decreased > free T4

Hypothyroidism

540. What are the most common etiologies of hypothyroidism?
   ➢ Primary (most common)
   ➢ Hashimoto's thyroiditis
   ➢ Radioactive iodine

> Radiation therapy

541. What type of reflexes would you expect in a patient with hypothyroidism?

> Delayed

542. What is the typical pattern of TSH and free T4 in subclinical hypothyroidism? Hypothyroidism?

> Subclinical hypothyroidism:
>   - Elevated TSH
>   - Normal free T4
> Hypothyroidism:
>   - Elevated TSH
>   - Decreased free T4

543. What is the first-line pharmacologic treatment for hypothyroidism?

> Levothyroxine

544. What antiarrhythmic medication is a common cause of secondary hypothyroidism?

> Amiodarone

545. What is the cause of myxedema crisis? What are the symptoms?

> Profound hypothyroidism
> Hypotension, hypoventilation, changes in mental status, and hypoglycemia

Hyperthyroidism

546. What is the utility of the radioactive iodine uptake (RAIU) scan?

> Helps differentiate causes of hyperthyroidism

547. What are the causes of diffuse RAIU?

> Toxic multinodular goiter

➤ Grave's disease

548. What are the causes of local RAIU?

➤ Functional adenoma

549. What is the RAIU pattern of thyroiditis?

➤ No RAIU

550. What are the common causes of hyperthyroidism?

➤ Grave's disease

➤ Single or multinodular goiter

➤ Thyroiditis

➤ TSH secreting pituitary tumor

551. What is the most common physical exam findings in Graves ophthalmopathy?

➤ Exophthalmos

552. What is a classic dermatologic complication of Graves disease-causing edema of the lower extremities?

➤ Pretibial myxedema

553. What is the first-line therapy for the treatment of palpitation due to hyperthyroidism?

➤ Beta-blockers

554. What are the two most common pharmacologic antithyroid agents?

➤ Methimazole

➤ Propylthiouracil (PTU)

555. What labs should be monitored while on PTU and methimazole due to their adverse side effects?

➤ Liver functions test

556. Which antithyroid agent should be used during the first trimester of pregnancy?

➤ PTU

Thyroiditis

557. What is the most common cause of painful thyroiditis?
> DeQuervain's (viral infection)

558. What thyroid antibody is commonly elevated in Hashimoto's thyroiditis?
> Antithyroid peroxidase (TPO)

559. What are the common causes of painless thyroiditis?
> Autoimmune
> Lymphocytic
> Postpartum
> Radiation

Diabetes Mellitus

Screening & Diagnosis

560. What are three primary methods used to screen for diabetes?
> Hemoglobin A1c, fasting plasma glucose, two-hour plasma glucose during a 75-gram oral glucose tolerance test

561. What is the ideal method to diagnose diabetes mellitus?
> Repeating testing of the same test on a different day or obtaining fasting plasma glucose and simultaneous hemoglobin A1c

562. What should you do if the two screening tests for diabetes are discordant?
> Repeat the test that gave a normal value

563. What glucose values for each of the three primary screening tests meet the criteria for the diagnosis of prediabetes?

➤ Two-hour oral glucose tolerance test: 140-190 mg/dL
➤ Hemoglobin A1c: 5.7-6.4%
➤ Impaired fasting glucose: 100-125 mg/dL

564. What glucose values for each of the three primary screening tests meet criteria for the diagnosis of diabetes?

➤ Two-hour oral glucose tolerance test: ≥200 mg/dL
➤ Hemoglobin A1c: ≥6.5%
➤ Impaired fasting glucose: ≥126 mg/dL

565. What are conditions that can result in a falsely low hemoglobin A1c and should prompt use of other tests for glycemic screening and/or monitoring?

➤ Conditions with an increase in red blood cell turnover and in turn, decrease the amount of glycosylated red blood cells (ie. hemolytic anemia, treatment with erythropoietin, chronic kidney disease)

566. When should patients with type 2 diabetes be screened for diabetic polyneuropathy?

➤ At the time of diagnosis and then yearly thereafter with a 10-gram monofilament

567. What is the most common distribution of diabetic neuropathy?

➤ Stocking-glove pattern

568. When should a patient with type 2 diabetes be screened for ocular complications of diabetes?

> At the time of diagnosis and then yearly thereafter with fundoscopic retinal exams

569. What are common ocular complications of diabetes mellitus?

> Diabetic retinopathy, diabetic macular edema, cataracts, and glaucoma

570. What are the common microvascular and macrovascular complications of long-standing diabetes?

> Microvascular complications: Microalbuminuria/proteinuria, retinopathy, polyneuropathy

> Macrovascular complications: Ischemic cardiovascular disease, ischemic cerebrovascular disease, peripheral vascular disease, chronic renal disease, erectile dysfunction

Treatment

571. What is the first line approach in the treatment of type 2 diabetes mellitus per the American Diabetes Association?

> Lifestyle modification (ie. diet, weight reduction, exercise) and metformin

572. What are the first line pharmacologic therapies for patients with type 2 diabetes mellitus and cardiovascular disease per the American Diabetes Association?

> GLP-1 receptor agonists (ie. liraglutide, dulaglutide, semaglutide, exenatide)

> SGLT2 inhibitors (ie. empagliflozin, dapagliflozin, canagliflozin)

573. When should insulin therapy be initiated in a person with type 2 diabetes?

> Fasting blood glucose: ≥250 mg/dL
> Hemoglobin A1c: >10%
> Consistent random blood glucose: >300 mg/dL
> Initial presentation of symptomatic diabetic ketoacidosis (DKA) (ie. weight loss, polydipsia, polyuria)

574. What are the treatment options for painful diabetic polyneuropathy?

> Amitriptyline, duloxetine, pregabalin, gabapentin, strict glycemic control

575. What is a common adverse effect of metformin that may decrease adherence to the medication?

> Diarrhea in a dose dependent manner

576. What is a potential adverse effect of metformin that commonly prompts discontinuation of the medication during an in-patient hospitalization?

> Lactic acidosis

577. What are the potential adverse effects of SGLT2 inhibitors?

> Dehydration, hypovolemia, euglycemic diabetes ketoacidosis (DKA), lower limb amputations, frequent UTIs, and GU fungal infections, Fournier's gangrene

578. What are common adverse effects of gabapentin and pregabalin?

> Peripheral edema, ataxia, dizziness, fatigue, drowsiness

579. When is metformin therapy contraindicated in patients with chronic kidney disease?

> eGFR <30 mL/min/1.73 m²

Diabetic Ketoacidosis (DKA)

580. What are common precipitants of diabetic ketoacidosis (DKA)?

> Infections, infarctions, alcohol and drug intoxication, nonadherence to insulin, pancreatitis

581. What is the pathophysiology of ketosis?

> Oxidation of fatty acids due to insulin deficiency which leads to increased substrates for ketogenesis by the liver

582. What is considered the "triad" of DKA?

> Anion gap metabolic acidosis
> Hyperglycemia
> Ketonemia

583. What differentiates DKA from the hyperosmolar hyperglycemic state (HHS)?

> Absence of keto acids in HHS

584. At what serum potassium should insulin infusion be delayed and aggressive electrolyte replacement be performed in a patient with DKA?

> <3.3 mEq/L

585. When should dextrose be added to the IV fluid regime in the treatment of DKA?

> Serum glucose <200 mg/dL

586. What is the IV fluid of choice in the initial treatment of DKA?

> 0.9% normal saline

587. What criteria should be met prior to discontinuation of the insulin infusion in the management of DKA?

> Normal serum anion gap
> Blood glucose <200 mg/dL
> Patient tolerating PO intake
> Venous pH >7.3, or serum bicarbonate >15 mEq/L

Disorders of the Adrenal Glands

Adrenal Insufficiency

588. What is the location of disease in primary adrenal insufficiency (AI)? In secondary AI?

> Primary: Adrenocortical disease (Addison's disease)
> Secondary: Pituitary gland

589. What are the etiologies of primary AI?

> Vascular (sepsis)
> Deposition disease (amyloidosis, sarcoidosis, hemochromatosis)
> Infection
> Autoimmune
> Drugs

590. What are the most common clinical manifestations of primary and secondary AI?

> Weakness, fatigue, orthostatic hypotension, anorexia, weight loss

591. What is the classic dermatologic manifestation of primary AI?

> Hyperpigmentation seen in mucous membranes, nipples, and creases

592. What levels of morning serum cortisol can effectively rule in AI? Rule out AI?

> Rules it in: <3 ug/dL
> Rules it out: >18 ug/dL

593. What is the most common diagnostic test to evaluate for AI?

> Cosyntropin stimulation test

594. What are two imaging studies to consider in the evaluation of AI?

> Pituitary MRI
> Abdominal CT to evaluate the adrenal glands

595. What is the management of acute AI (adrenal crisis)?

> IV fluids
> IV hydrocortisone

596. What must be ruled out in the workup of a patient with an incidentally found adrenal adenoma? What else should be worked up in patients with hypertension?

> Cushing's syndrome and pheochromocytoma
> Workup of hyperaldosteronism

Pheochromocytoma

597. What are the clinical manifestations of pheochromocytomas?

> Hypertension
> Headaches

> Palpitations
> Perspiration

598. What is the serum diagnostic study of choice for pheochromocytoma?
> Plasma free metanephrines

599. What is the appropriate treatment algorithm for pheochromocytoma?
> Alpha blockade first
> Beta blockade prior to performing surgery

Hypercortisolism

600. What are classic physical manifestations of hypercortisolism?
> Dorsocervical fat pad
> Rounded facies
> Central obesity with extremity wasting
> Striae
> Spontaneous bruising

601. What are the three screening tests to evaluate hypercortisolism?
> 24-hour urine free cortisol
> 1 mg dexamethasone suppression test
> 11 PM salivary cortisol x 3 samples

602. What is the difference between Cushing's syndrome and Cushing's disease? What is the most common cause of each?
> Syndrome: Cortisol excess
  - Exogenous glucocorticoids
> Disease: Pituitary ACTH hypersecretion causing Cushing's syndrome

- Pituitary adenoma

603. What are the two other etiologies of hypercortisolism?

> Adrenal tumor
> Ectopic ACTH
  - Small cell lung cancer, carcinoid, etc.

Hyperaldosteronism

604. What are the causes of primary hyperaldosteronism? Secondary hyperaldosteronism?

> Primary: Adrenal disorder and renin independent (ie. adenoma, carcinoma, adrenal hyperplasia)
> Secondary: Aldosterone is renin dependent (ie. CHF, cirrhosis, nephrotic syndrome, diuretics, Bartter's and Gitelman's syndromes)

605. What are the clinical manifestations of hyperaldosteronism?

> Hypertension
> Weakness
> Headaches
> Hypokalemia (may be normal)

606. What is the screening test of choice for the evaluation of hyperaldosteronism?

> 8 AM plasma aldosterone : renin ratio
  - >20 suggestive of primary hyperaldosteronism

607. What is the confirmatory test of choice for hyperaldosteronism?

> Sodium suppression test (oral sodium loading over three days)

Disorders of Calcium Homeostasis

General

608. What hormone is the key regulator of calcium and phosphate homeostasis?
    ➢ Parathyroid hormone (PTH)
609. What is the main calcium binding protein?
    ➢ Albumin
610. Serum calcium is a measurement of what?
    ➢ Both bound and unbound calcium
        ▪ Physiologically active calcium is free (unbound)

Hypercalcemia

611. What is the most common cause of hypercalcemia?
    ➢ Hyperparathyroidism secondary to an adenoma
612. What are common manifestations of hypercalcemia?
    ➢ Polyuria, hypovolemia, encephalopathy, fractures, nephrolithiasis, abdominal pain, nausea, and vomiting
613. What malignancies classically cause an increase in hypercalcemia? What is the identifiable peptide associated with this hypercalcemia?
    ➢ Squamous cell, breast, and renal cell cancers
    ➢ Parathyroid hormone-related peptide (PTHrP)
614. What are the classic causes of Vitamin D excess causing hypercalcemia?
    ➢ Sarcoidosis
    ➢ Tuberculosis

615. What diuretic can classically lead to hypercalcemia?

> Thiazides

616. What is the serum albumin-corrected calcium that is considered mild hypercalcemia? Moderate? Severe?

> Mild: <12 mg/dL
> Moderate: 12-14 mg/dL
> Severe: >14 mg/dL

617. What is the treatment for patients with mild hypercalcemia? Moderate? Severe?

> Mild: Avoid precipitating drug and conservative management
> Moderate: IV saline and bisphosphonates if patient is significantly symptomatic
> Severe: Aggressive volume expansion, calcitonin, bisphosphonates, and zoledronic acid

Hypocalcemia

618. What are clinical manifestations of hypocalcemia?

> Osteomalacia, osteitis fibrosa cystica, perioral paresthesias, cramps, irritability, depression, psychosis

619. What are the causes of hypocalcemia with low PTH?

> Surgical resection of parathyroid hormone
> Autoimmune disease

620. What are the causes of hypocalcemia with high PTH?

> Chronic kidney disease
> Impaired PTH action

Endocrinology

- ➤ Vitamin D deficiency
- ➤ Hyperphosphatemia
- ➤ Acute pancreatitis
- ➤ Sepsis
- ➤ Malignancy

5

GASTROENTEROLOGY

Gastrointestinal Bleed

Upper GI Bleed (UGIB) & Esophageal Varices

621. What is the most common cause of an upper GI bleeding (UGIB) in patients in North America? What are the other causes of UGIB?

> ➢ Peptic ulcer
> ➢ Variceal bleeding, gastritis, duodenitis, gastropathy, Mallory-Weiss tears, erosive esophagitis, and angioectasias

622. What are the two most common etiologies of peptic ulcers?

> ➢ NSAIDs and Helicobacter pylori

623. What is a Dieulafoy lesion?

> ➢ A gastric artery that has eroded into the mucosa and can cause a massive UGIB

624. What is the beneficial mechanism of action of PPI therapy in the acute setting in patients with UGIB?

> ➢ Increase gastric pH to allow platelet aggregation

625. What class of beta-blockers are used in the treatment of primary prevention of esophageal varices?

> ➢ Nonselective beta-blockers

626. What is the pharmacologic therapy for an acute variceal bleed?

> ➢ Octreotide IV infusion and ceftriaxone

627. How long do you continue PPIs after endoscopic therapy in a patient with UGIB due to PUD or an ulcer with stigmata of recent hemorrhage?

> ➢ Continue PPI infusion post endotherapy for 72 hours prior to converting to oral PPIs

628. What is the mechanism of action of nonselective beta-blockers in the use of primary prevention of esophageal variceal bleeds?

  ➢ Decreased cardiac output (B1 adrenergic blockade) and B2 adrenergic blockade leading to unopposed alpha-adrenergic splanchnic vasoconstriction

629. What medication has been shown to decrease mortality in acute esophageal variceal hemorrhage?

  ➢ Antibiotics
    ▪ Most commonly ceftriaxone

630. What artery is directly posterior to the posterior duodenal wall and can lead to massive UGIB?

  ➢ Gastroduodenal artery

631. Administration of proton pump inhibitors in the setting of an UGIB prevents what?

  ➢ In the pre-endoscopic phase, they decrease the need for endoscopy therapy but do not decrease mortality, length of stay, or need for blood transfusions
  ➢ For patients with high-risk stigmata and post-endoscopic therapy, high-dose continuous PPI infusions do decrease bleeding and mortality compared with placebo or H2 receptor antagonists

632. What is the benefit of administering a prokinetic agent such as metoclopramide in the setting of a UGIB?

  ➢ Decrease the need for a repeat endoscopy

- They do not decrease the length of stay or mortality

Gastric Antral Vascular Ectasias (GAVE)

633. What is the pathognomonic endoscopic finding of gastric antral vascular ectasias (GAVE)?
  ➢ Watermelon stomach

634. What comorbidities are classically associated with GAVE?
  ➢ Cirrhosis and systemic sclerosis

Lower GI Bleed (LGIB)

635. What is the anatomical landmark that defines an upper vs lower GI bleed (LGIB)?
  ➢ Ligament of Treitz

636. What is the most common cause of LGIB? What are the other common causes of LGIB?
  ➢ Most common: Diverticulosis
  ➢ Other common causes: Malignancy, infectious, inflammatory, ischemic colitis, angioectasia, hemorrhoids, anal fissure, radiation proctopathy, stercoral colitis, post-polypectomy

Small Bowel Disease

Celiac Disease

637. What signs and symptoms should prompt testing for celiac disease?
  ➢ Signs of malabsorption such as diarrhea, weight loss, steatorrhea, bloating, and postprandial

abdominal pain or findings such as early
osteoporosis and iron-deficiency anemia

638. What is the recommended initial screening test for celiac disease?

> Anti-tissue transglutaminase (TTG) immunoglobulin A (IgA) as well as a total IgA (evaluate for IgA deficiency)

639. What diet should a patient be on prior to diagnostic serologic testing for evaluation of celiac disease?

> Gluten-containing diet

640. What is the confirmatory test of choice for a positive celiac screening test?

> Small bowel biopsy

641. What is the classic finding on endoscopy in a patient with celiac disease?

> Villous atrophy/blunting with increased intraepithelial lymphocytes and crypt hyperplasia

642. What are other causes of duodenal villous atrophy?

> Tropical sprue, Whipple's disease, Crohn's disease, collagenous sprue, infections (ie. Giardiasis or H. pylori), graft versus host disease, acquired immune deficiency syndrome enteropathy, autoimmune enteropathy, common variable immunodeficiency, olmesartan

643. What diet should patients with celiac disease adhere to?

> Gluten free diet

Gastroenterology

Whipple's Disease

644. What are the classic symptoms of Whipple's Disease?
> Arthralgia, diarrhea, weight loss, abdominal pain, and neurologic symptoms

645. What is the first line therapy for Whipple's Disease?
> Initial IV antibiotics (ie. ceftriaxone, penicillin) followed by trimethoprim-sulfamethoxazole (Bactrim) for 1 year of maintenance therapy

646. What is the classic histologic finding of Whipple's disease?
> Periodic acid-Schiff (PAS) positive macrophages in the lamina propria

Systemic Scleroderma

647. What are common GI manifestations of systemic scleroderma?
> Esophageal dysmotility, small bowel dysmotility, SIBO, malabsorption

Small Bowel Enteropathy

648. What ACEi is commonly associated with causing small bowel enteropathy?
> Olmesartan

Inflammatory Bowel Disease (IBD)

General

649. What are the common types of inflammatory bowel disease (IBD)?

> Ulcerative colitis
> Crohn's disease
> Microscopic colitis

650. What are the classic ocular manifestations most commonly associated with IBD?

> Uveitis, scleritis, and episcleritis

651. What are the classic dermatologic manifestations most commonly associated with IBD?

> Pyoderma gangrenosum and erythema nodosum

652. What is the typical age onset of ulcerative colitis and Crohn's disease?

> 15-30 years old with another peak at 50-70 years old

653. When should the first surveillance colonoscopy be performed in patients with newly diagnosed ulcerative colitis or Crohn's disease with extensive colonic involvement?

> 8-10 years after diagnosis

654. What pharmacologic therapy class should be considered for a severe exacerbation of IBD?

> Corticosteroids
>> ▪ IV steroids commonly used for inpatients
>> ▪ Oral steroids commonly used in outpatients

655. What should be excluded in all patients presenting with signs and symptoms of a IBD flare?

➢ Superimposed infections (ie. C. difficile) or other enteric infections

656. In a person with ileocolonic resection what can be a common noninfectious and noninflammatory cause of diarrhea?

➢ Bile acid diarrhea

657. Patients taking TNF-alpha antagonists are at increased risk for what type of skin cancer?

➢ Melanoma

Microscopic Colitis

658. What are the two types of microscopic colitis?

➢ Collagenous
➢ Lymphocytic

659. What is the common clinical manifestation of microscopic colitis?

➢ Insidious or acute onset of non-bloody watery diarrhea common in the elderly

660. Common pharmacologic causes of microscopic colitis?

➢ NSAIDs, ACEi, statins, SSRIs, PPIs

Crohn's Disease

661. What are the most common symptom of Crohn's disease?

➢ Diarrhea, weight loss, abdominal pain, hematochezia

662. What is the classic endoscopic colonic disease distribution of Crohn's disease?

> Patchy areas of inflammation that appear to "skip" throughout the colon and with sparing of the rectum

663. How does Crohn's disease affect the mucosa and submucosal tissues as compared to ulcerative colitis?

> Crohn's disease classically has transmural involvement of both the mucosa and submucosal tissues
  - Ulcerative colitis is limited to the mucosa

664. What is the only FDA approved biologic for the treatment of fistulizing Crohn's disease?

> Infliximab

Ulcerative Colitis

665. Which extraintestinal system is most frequently affected by ulcerative colitis?

> Musculoskeletal (ie. arthropathy)

666. What are the three anatomic subtypes of ulcerative colitis?

> Proctitis (limited to the rectum)
> Left-sided ulcerative colitis/proctosigmoiditis (distal to the splenic flexure to the rectum)
> Extensive colitis/pancolitis (disease that extends more proximal to the splenic flexure)
  - Includes the transverse colon, ascending colon, and/or rectum

Gastroenterology

Colorectal Cancer

General

667. When should patients with a family history of colorectal cancer in a first degree relative undergo colorectal cancer screening?

> Age 40 or 10 years prior to the earliest age of diagnosis of the family member (whichever comes first)

Familial Adenomatous Polyposis (FAP)

668. Development of hundreds to thousands of adenomatous polyps in the lower GI tract should raise concern for what?

> Familial adenomatous polyposis (FAP)

669. What is the inheritance pattern of FAP?

> Autosomal dominant

670. A germline mutation in what gene is responsible for FAP?

> Adenomatous polyposis coli (APC), when mutated, leads to the accumulation of beta-catenin, activation of the Wnt signaling pathway, and uncontrolled cell growth

671. What is the standard of care in the management of colorectal polyposis due to FAP?

> Proctocolectomy

672. What are risk factors for FAP?

> First degree relative with FAP and patients with >10 cumulative colorectal adenomas or any

number of adenomas with extracolonic features of FAP

673. What are extracolonic features of FAP?

> Duodenal/ampullary adenomas, desmoid tumors, papillary thyroid cancer, congenital hypertrophy of retinal pigment epithelium, epidermal cysts, or osteomas

Gardner Syndrome

674. Gardner syndrome characteristically has what intestinal and extraintestinal lesions?

> FAP, osteomas, dental abnormalities, desmoid tumors, and fibromas

Diarrhea & Constipation
General

675. What is the first line therapy for opioid induced constipation?

> Osmotic laxatives
  - If those fail then Mu-opioid receptor antagonist such as methylnaltrexone

676. In a patient with chronic diarrhea or constipation what hormone should be checked?

> TSH

Bile Acid Malabsorption

677. What are the signs and symptoms of bile acid malabsorption?

> Diarrhea (hallmark), fecal urgency, abdominal pain, bloating

678. What surgical procedure is a risk factor for the development of bile acid malabsorption?

> Ileal resection (think a patient with Crohn's disease who underwent ileal resection)

Irritable Bowel Syndrome (IBS)

679. Linaclotide is used in the treatment of what type of irritable bowel syndrome (IBS)?

> Constipation predominant

680. What are the criteria for the diagnosis of IBS?

> Abdominal pain at least 1 day/week for the past three months and at least two of the following:
  - Change in stool frequency
  - Change in stool form
  - Changes related to defecation

Small Intestinal Bacterial Overgrowth (SIBO)

681. What is the etiology of small intestinal bacterial overgrowth (SIBO)?

> Functional or motility disorder leading to colonic bacterial overgrowth in the small intestine

682. What is the most common presenting symptom of SIBO?

> Bloating, followed by diarrhea, increased flatulence, and abdominal discomfort

683. How do you establish the diagnosis of SIBO?

> Hydrogen breath test or jejunal aspirate

684. What is the first-line pharmacotherapy of SIBO?

➤ Antibiotics such as rifaximin

Dumping Syndrome

685. What is dumping or rapid gastric emptying syndrome?

➤ Rapid emptying of food into the small intestine causes rapid fluid shifts due to hyperosmolality of the food leading to abdominal pain, bloating, and diarrhea

686. What type of surgery is a risk factor for dumping syndrome?

➤ Bariatric surgery

Pancreas

Acute Pancreatitis

687. What are the diagnostic criteria for acute pancreatitis?

➤ Must have at least 2 of the following:
  ▪ Elevated lipase $\geq$ 3x upper limit of normal
  ▪ Characteristic pain of pancreatitis
  ▪ Imaging findings consistent with pancreatitis

688. What imaging test should be performed in all patients with acute pancreatitis?

➤ Transabdominal ultrasound

689. What is the most critical first step in the management of acute pancreatitis?

➤ IV fluid hydration

690. What type of IV fluid is recommended as first line therapy for resuscitation in acute pancreatitis?

➢ Lactated Ringers

691. When should enteral feeding be initiated in a patient with acute pancreatitis?

➢ As soon as the patient is able to tolerate it as early enteral feeding is associated with less comorbidities

Insulinoma

692. What is the most common pancreatic endocrine tumor?

➢ Insulinoma

Ascending Cholangitis

693. What is Charcot's triad?

➢ RUQ pain, fever, and jaundice concerning ascending cholangitis

694. In a patient with ascending cholangitis what procedure should be performed urgently?

➢ ERCP

Pancreatic Adenocarcinoma

695. What is the most well-established risk factor for pancreatic adenocarcinoma?

➢ Cigarette smoking

Autoimmune Pancreatitis

696. What is the first-line treatment for autoimmune pancreatitis?

➢ Glucocorticoids

Drug Induced Pancreatitis

697. What common medications are associated with drug induced pancreatitis?

> Azathioprine, sulfonamides, valproic acid, estrogen

Hypertriglyceridemia Induced Pancreatitis

698. What serum triglyceride level is required for the diagnosis of hypertriglyceridemia induced pancreatitis?

> >1000 mg/dL

699. What are the two main treatment modalities for hypertriglyceridemia induced pancreatitis??

> Plasmapheresis and insulin

Infectious Enteritis & Colitis

700. What is the first-line therapy for C. difficile infection?

> PO vancomycin or fidaxomicin

701. What two organisms classically can present with right lower quadrant pain and can be confused for appendicitis?

> Yersinia enterocolitica and Campylobacter jejuni

702. What are the risk factors for Yersinia enterocolitica infections?

> Consuming raw or undercooked pork, untreated water, and hemochromatosis

703. What are the most common presenting signs and symptoms of Strongyloides stercoralis infection?

> Waxing and waning diarrhea, abdominal pain,
> eosinophilia, rash, and pulmonary symptoms that
> can persist for years

704. What is the first-line treatment for Strongyloides
stercoralis?

> Ivermectin

705. What is the first-line therapy for Giardiasis?

> Tinidazole

706. What tapeworm can cause a Vitamin B12
deficiency?

> Diphyllobothrium latum

707. What food is the most common cause of Shigella
toxin-producing E. coli (STEC) infections?

> Undercooked ground beef, contaminated food,
> raw food, and raw milk

708. What is the first-line therapy for STEC?

> Supportive with the aggressive replacement of
> electrolytes, rehydration, monitoring of kidney
> function and thrombocytopenia

709. The use of antibiotics in patients with STEC is
associated with an increased risk of what?

> Development of hemolytic uremic syndrome

710. What is the most common cause of foodborne
gastroenteritis in the USA?

> Norovirus infection

711. What gram-negative bacteria is the leading cause
of shellfish associated deaths in the USA?

> Vibrio vulnificus

712. Patients with a history of what liver pathology are
at increased risk of severe vibrio vulnificus infection?

> Cirrhosis

713. What is the most common symptom of a pinworm infection?

> Perianal itching

714. What are the most commonly infected colonic segments in patients with Entamoeba histolytica?

> Cecum and ascending colon

715. What is the treatment of choice in an immunocompetent adult with cyclosporiasis?

> Trimethoprim-sulfamethoxazole

Liver

End-Stage Liver Disease

716. What is the Model for End-stage Liver Disease (MELD)?

> Prognostic scoring model for prediction mortality related to cirrhosis over the subsequent 3 months

717. What lab values are used to calculate the MELD score?

> INR, serum bilirubin, serum creatinine
> MELD-Na also incorporates sodium

Varices

718. In patients with cirrhosis, upper endoscopy is recommended to screen for what?

> Varices

719. What are the most common risk factors for variceal hemorrhage?

Gastroenterology

> Variceal size (larger more likely), red wale sign
seen on endoscopy, and decompensated cirrhosis

720. In a patient with varices who have never bled what
are the two approaches to primary prophylaxis?

> Variceal banding or non-selective beta-blockers

Spontaneous Bacterial Peritonitis

721. What is the ascitic fluid neutrophil count required
for the diagnosis of spontaneous bacterial peritonitis
(SBP)?

> $>250/mm^3$

722. What oral medications used for reflux is associated
with an increased risk of SBP?

> PPIs

723. Should patients who survived a first case of SBP
receive lifelong prophylaxis for prevention of
recurrence of SBP?

> Yes

Hepatic Encephalopathy

724. What are the most common causes of acute
hepatic encephalopathy in patients with cirrhosis?

> Infections, GI bleeding, constipation, opioid use,
over diuresis

725. In patients with persistent or recurrent hepatic
encephalopathy what antibiotic should be added to
lactulose?

> Rifaximin

Ascites & Cirrhosis

726. What diuretic combination is used in the management of ascites due to cirrhosis?
   ➢ Furosemide and spironolactone

727. What is the preferred ratio of furosemide and spironolactone
   ➢ 40:100 and titrate up per that ratio

728. What should be the initial laboratory investigation in all patients with ascites?
   ➢ Ascitic fluid cell count and differential, albumin, culture, total protein, and calculating the SAAG ratio

729. What is the SAAG ratio? What do the values indicate?
   ➢ Serum albumin minus ascites ratio
      ▪ SAAG >1.1 g/dL suggests portal hypertension

730. What is the differential diagnosis for ascites other than cirrhosis?
   ➢ Nephrotic syndrome, tuberculosis, heart failure, malignancy

731. What is the recommended diet for patients with cirrhosis?
   ➢ Dietary sodium restrictions of <2000 mg/day

732. What is considered refractory ascites?
   ➢ Unresponsive to maximum dosing spironolactone/furosemide (400 mg/160 mg), unresponsive to sodium restricted diet, or rapid recurrence of ascites after therapeutic paracentesis

733. When is post paracentesis albumin infusion indicated?

> Large volume paracentesis of ≥5 liters
>   ▪ Order 6-8 grams of albumin per liter removed

Hepatorenal Syndrome

734. What are the major criteria for the diagnosis of type 1 hepatorenal syndrome (HRS)?

> Cirrhosis with ascites
> Serum creatinine > 1.5 mg/dL
> No improvement in serum creatinine after 2 days with diuretic withdrawal and volume expansion with albumin
> Absence of shock
> Absence of nephrotoxic drugs
> Absence of abnormal renal ultrasonography

735. What is the difference between type 1 and type 2 HRS?

> Type 1: Rapidly progressive reduction in kidney function with doubling of the initial serum creatinine to a level >2.5 mg/dL or a 50% reduction of the initial 24-hour creatinine clearance in <2 weeks
> Type 2: Less rapidly progressive disease

736. What is the initial treatment of type 1 HRS?

> Albumin infusion with octreotide and midodrine

Hepatic Hydrothorax

737. What is the first-line therapy for hepatic hydrothorax?

> Dietary sodium restrictions and diuretic therapy

Acute Liver Failure

738. What is the definition of acute liver failure (ALF)?
> Coagulation abnormalities (INR ≥1.5) and any degree of mental alteration in patients without cirrhosis and illness duration <26 weeks

739. What is the leading cause of ALF in the United States?
> Acetaminophen toxicity

740. If acetaminophen ingestion is suspected to be the cause of ALF what gastrointestinal decontaminant can be given orally if it is within 4 hours of ingestion?
> Activated charcoal

741. What is the antidote to acetaminophen poisoning?
> N-acetylcysteine (NAC)

Viral Hepatitis

742. Hepatitis delta only occurs in patients with what superimposed viral infection?
> Hepatitis B

743. What is the route of transmission of hepatitis A?
> Fecal-oral route

744. Which hepatotropic virus commonly found in the U.S. is the only virus not preventable through vaccination?
> Hepatitis C

745. Which hepatotropic virus is associated with porphyria cutanea tarda?
> Hepatitis C

746. What is the most likely diagnosis in a patient with hepatitis C with arthralgias, weakness, and purpura?

> Mixed cryoglobulinemia

747. In patients with chronic hepatitis B virus, liver imaging surveillance is recommended to identify development of what malignancy?

> Hepatocellular carcinoma

748. What are the common modes of transmission of hepatitis B and C?

> IV drug use, tattoos and body piercings, vertical transmission, blood transfusions, sex

Alcoholic Hepatitis

749. What clinical score can be useful in determining whether an episode of alcoholic hepatitis is severe?

> Maddrey Discriminant Function ($\geq$32) or MELD score is >20

750. What is the treatment of severe acute alcoholic hepatitis? What is the major contraindication to this treatment?

> Prednisolone and abstinence from alcohol

> Contraindication to prednisolone: Infections

751. What clinical model should be used to assess response to prednisolone therapy in alcoholic hepatitis?

> Lille model

752. What noninvasive imaging modality is useful to assess the stages of hepatic fibrosis?

> Elastography

Autoimmune Hepatitis

753. What is the characteristic histologic abnormality seen in autoimmune hepatitis (AIH)?
  ➤ Lymphoplasmacytic interface hepatitis
    ▪ Interface hepatitis is the histologic hallmark of AIH

754. Which sex has the higher predominance of AIH?
  ➤ Females

755. What are the conventional autoantibodies associated with AIH?
  ➤ Antinuclear antibodies (ANA), anti-liver kidney microsome type 1 (LKM1), and smooth muscle antibodies (SMA)

756. What autoantibodies are associated with each type of AIH?
  ➤ Type 1 AIH: ANA and/or SMA
  ➤ Type 2 AIH: Anti-LKM1

757. Do patients with suspected AIH require a liver biopsy?
  ➤ Yes, the diagnosis of AIH cannot be made without a liver biopsy

758. What 2 other autoimmune diseases should be screened for in patients with AIH at initial diagnosis?
  ➤ Celiac and thyroid disease

759. What is the first line therapy in patients with AIH?
  ➤ Prednisone alone or prednisone in combination with azathioprine

760. What is the minimum duration of therapy in AIH?
  ➤ 2 years before attempts at treatment withdrawal

Hemochromatosis

761. What is the most common genetic mutation of the HFE gene in patients with hemochromatosis?
  ➤ C282Y

762. What is another common regulatory mutation of the HFE gene?
  ➤ H63D

763. What is the principal iron regulatory hormone?
  ➤ Hepcidin

764. What is the treatment of patients with hemochromatosis and iron overload?
  ➤ Weekly phlebotomy

Nonalcoholic Fatty Liver Disease

765. What are common conditions that are high risk factors for the development of nonalcoholic fatty liver disease (NAFLD)?
  ➤ Obesity, type 2 diabetes, dyslipidemia, polycystic ovarian syndrome

Primary Biliary Cholangitis (PBC)

766. What is the hallmark serologic antibody in primary biliary cholangitis (PBC)?
  ➤ Antimitochondrial antibody (AMA)

767. What is the initial drug of choice in the treatment of PBC?
  ➤ Ursodeoxycholic acid (UDCA)

768. What is the most common symptom in patients with PBC?
  ➤ Fatigue

Primary Sclerosing Cholangitis (PSC)

769. What is the characteristic pattern of disease in patients with primary sclerosing cholangitis (PSC)?

> Inflammation and fibrosis of **both** intrahepatic and extrahepatic bile ducts

770. Do testing of autoantibodies have a role in the diagnosis of PSC?

> No, as a wide range of autoantibodies can be detected in the serum of patients with PSC

771. What is the characteristic pattern of PSC as seen on MRI?

> Bile ducts showing multifocal strictures and segmental dilations

772. If a person is found to have primary sclerosing cholangitis (PSC), when should they obtain a colonoscopy?

> At diagnosis and every year thereafter

773. Why should a person with PSC and concomitant IBD undergo yearly colonoscopies?

> PSC is the most consistent risk factor for colorectal cancer in patients with IBD

Wilson Disease

774. What is the abnormal gene in Wilson disease?

> Absent or reduced function in ATP7B

775. What is the consequence of an absent or redacted function in ATP7B?

> Decreased hepatocellular excretion of copper and therefore an accumulation and injury in the liver

776. What is the classic ocular manifestation of Wilson disease?

> Kayser-Fleischer rings

777. What are common psychiatric features in patients with Wilson disease?

> Depression, neurotic behavior, personality changes

778. What are common neurologic features in patients with Wilson disease?

> Movement disorders, pseudobulbar palsy, migraine headache, insomnia, dysarthria

779. What urine testing should be obtained in all patients with suspected Wilson disease?

> Urine 24-hour excretion of copper

780. What is the initial treatment of choice for symptomatic patients with Wilson disease?

> Chelating agents such as D-penicillamine or trientine

Miscellaneous

General

781. In a patient with a history of atrial fibrillation who presents with acute abdominal pain out of proportion to the physical examination, what should be suspected?

> Acute mesenteric ischemia

782. What should be suspected in a patient with superficial abdominal wall pain with tenderness to light palpation?

> Anterior cutaneous nerve entrapment syndrome and shingles

783. In a patient with ulcerations of the mucosa, genitalia, and small bowel, what disease should be suspected?

> Bechet's disease

784. What is the most common metabolic cause of gastroparesis?

> Diabetes mellitus

785. What promotility pharmacologic therapy is approved by the FDA for the management of gastroparesis?

> Metoclopramide

786. What are common and classic causes of pill induced esophagitis?

> Doxycycline, bisphosphonates, potassium chloride

787. What is the classic finding on barium swallow in achalasia?

> "Bird's beak" esophagus

Eosinophilic Esophagitis

788. What are the classic esophageal findings found on endoscopy that are suggestive of eosinophilic esophagitis?

> Trachealization and linear furrows in the esophagus

789. How many eosinophils are required to be seen on microscopy for the diagnosis of eosinophilic esophagitis?

> At least 15

Gastroenterology

H. pylori

790. What are the ways to test for H. pylori infections?
    ➢ Stool antigen testing, urease breath testing, and biopsy
791. What pharmacological therapeutic combinations are first line therapy for H. pylori with low risk of resistance?
    ➢ Triple therapy: Proton pump inhibitor and two antibiotics
792. Should H. pylori eradication testing be performed?
    ➢ Yes
        ▪ The patient should be off of PPIs for at least 2 weeks

Esophageal Candidiasis

793. What are risk factors for esophageal candidiasis?
    ➢ Diabetes mellitus, HIV-AIDS, immunosuppressive states, and corticosteroids
794. What is the first line therapy for esophageal candidiasis?
    ➢ Fluconazole

6

HEMATOLOGY

Anemia

Non-Hemolytic Anemias

795. In iron deficiency anemia, what changes would you expect in serum iron, ferritin, TIBC, and transferrin saturation?

> Iron: Decreased
> Ferritin: Decreased
> TIBC: Increased
> Transferrin saturation: Decreased (<10%)

796. In anemia of chronic disease, what changes would you expect in serum iron, ferritin, TIBC, and transferrin saturation?

> Iron: Decreased
> Ferritin: Increased
> TIBC: Decreased
> Transferrin saturation: Decreased/normal

797. What two potential etiologies should be evaluated for first when working up a patient with iron deficiency anemia?

> GI blood loss
> Menstrual blood loss

798. If iron deficiency anemia is not caused by blood loss, what other etiologies should be considered?

> Malabsorption
> Poor iron intake (i.e. vegetarians)

799. In a patient with macrocytic anemia, what nutritional deficiencies should be evaluated for?

> Folate
> Vitamin B12

800. If Vitamin B12 is low-normal, what additional tests should you perform to confirm Vitamin B12 deficiency?

> Methylmalonic acid
> Homocysteine levels

801. What autoimmune disorder is associated with Vitamin B12 deficiency? How can it be evaluated for serologically?

> Pernicious anemia
> Anti-IF antibodies

802. In patients with chronic alcohol use, what hematologic abnormality is often seen?

> Macrocytic anemia

803. What two nutrient deficiencies are the most common causes of anemia in pregnancy?

> Iron
> Folate

804. What type of anemia does lead poisoning cause?

> Sideroblastic anemia

805. What finding is seen on a peripheral blood smear in a patient with sideroblastic anemia?

> Basophilic stippling

806. In aplastic anemia, what cell lines are involved?

> All of them (RBC, WBC, and platelets)

807. Patients with aplastic anemia at increased risk for developing what two hematologic disorders?

> Acute leukemia
> Myelodysplastic syndrome

808. What is the treatment of aplastic anemia?

> Withdrawal of offending agents (if possible)

> Cyclosporine or antithymocyte globulin are first line
> Allogeneic hematopoietic stem cell transplant (HSCT) is potentially curative

Hemolytic Anemias

809. What labs are obtained when evaluating a patient with suspected hemolysis?

> LDH
> Haptoglobin
> Indirect bilirubin
> Reticulocyte count
> Coombs test

810. What enzyme deficiency would you suspect in a patient who develops new onset hemolytic anemia two weeks after starting Bactrim?

> Glucose-6-phosphate dehydrogenase (G6PD) deficiency

811. What are the characteristic findings on peripheral blood smear for patients with hemolysis due to G6PD deficiency?

> Bite cells

812. What diagnosis should be considered in a patient with hemolytic anemia, thrombocytopenia, and bloody diarrhea?

> Hemolytic uremic syndrome (HUS)

813. What pathogen is the most common etiology of HUS?

> E. coli O157:H7

814. What enzyme is reduced, either through enzyme deficiency or inhibition, in a patient with thrombotic thrombocytopenic purpura (TTP)?

> ADAMTS13

815. What is the classic pentad for a patient with TTP-HUS?

> Hemolytic anemia
> Thrombocytopenia
> Fever
> Renal failure
> Altered mental status

816. What is the treatment for a patient diagnosed with TTP?

> Emergent plasma exchange
> Steroids
> Refractory cases: Rituximab and bortezomib

817. What is seen on a peripheral blood smear for a patient with warm autoimmune hemolytic anemia?

> Spherocytes

818. What is the test to confirm warm autoimmune hemolytic anemia? What is the first line treatment?

> Direct Coombs test
> Steroids

819. What is the treatment for cold autoimmune hemolytic anemia?

> Cold avoidance
> Rituximab
> Warmed packed RBCs prior to transfusion
> Plasmapheresis

Hemoglobinopathies

Sickle Cell

820. How are sickle cell syndromes diagnosed?
> ➢ Hemoglobin electrophoresis

821. What is the treatment for a vasoocclusive crisis (VOC)?
> ➢ Hydration
> ➢ Supplemental oxygen if hypoxic
> ➢ Pain control
> ➢ Treat inciting event (i.e. antibiotics if infection)

822. What are the indications for exchange transfusion in sickle cell anemia?
> ➢ Acute stroke
> ➢ Acute coronary syndrome
> ➢ Fat embolism
> ➢ Acute chest syndrome

823. What medication is used to prevent VOC?
> ➢ Hydroxyurea

824. What treatment can be curative for sickle cell?
> ➢ Stem cell transplant

825. In sickle cells patients, what infection can trigger a pure red cell aplasia?
> ➢ Parvovirus B-19

Alpha & Beta Thalassemias

826. What is seen on hemoglobin electrophoresis for a patient with alpha thalassemia?
> ➢ Normal (~95% HbA, ~5% HbA2)

827. What is seen on hemoglobin electrophoresis in a patient with beta thalassemia?

> Elevated HbA2 and fetal hemoglobin

Hemostasis & Coagulation

General

828. What is the difference between primary and secondary hemostasis failure?

> Primary: A problem with platelet aggregation or platelet plug formation
> Secondary: Issues with tissue factor and the coagulation cascade

829. What signs and symptoms are characteristic of primary hemostasis failure?

> Epistaxis
> Gingival bleeding
> Easy bruising
> Menorrhagia

830. What findings are characteristic of secondary hemostasis pathology?

> Hemarthroses
> Intramuscular bleeding

831. How does a mixing study help to differentiate the etiology of a bleeding disorder in a patient with a prolonged PT or PTT?

> If the PT/PTT corrects in a mixing study, it suggests a factor deficiency
> If the PT/PTT does NOT correct, particularly with incubation, it suggests the presence of an inhibitor

832. What coagulation factors are Vitamin K dependent?
> Factors II, VII, IX, X
> Proteins C and S

833. What is the mechanism of action for heparin?
> Antithrombin III activator

834. What is the mechanism of action for coumadin?
> Inhibitor of synthesis of Vitamin K dependent clotting factors (II, VII, IX, X, Proteins C and S) by functionally depleting Vitamin K reserves

835. In what underlying protein deficiency is a patient at risk for warfarin skin necrosis?
> Protein C deficiency

836. In Caucasians, what is the most common hereditary etiology of thrombophilia?
> Factor V Leiden mutation

837. Should DVT prophylaxis be ordered for a patient with cirrhosis who is admitted for pneumonia, has an INR 2.1, and no signs of active bleeding?
> Yes, even though his INR is elevated, cirrhotics are not "auto-anticoagulated"

838. When should an IVC filter be placed?
> When a patient has an acute pelvic or proximal leg DVT and cannot be anticoagulated due to active bleeding or is at very high risk of bleeding

Hemophilia

839. What factors are deficient in Hemophilia A and B?
> Hemophilia A: Factor VIII
> Hemophilia B: Factor IX

840. Why are Hemophilia A and B seen mostly in men?
> X-Linked disorders

841. What medication can be given in to a patient with Hemophilia A before minor procedures to minimize bleeding?
> Desmopressin

Von Willebrand Disease

842. What is the role of von Willebrand factor (vWF)?
> It adheres platelets to injured vessels and acts as a carrier for factor VIII

843. How common is von Willebrand Disease?
> Affects 1% of the general population
  ▪ Most common inherited bleeding disorder

844. What medications can be used to treat minor bleeding or to minimize bleeding prophylactically (preoperative) in patients with von Willebrand Disease?
> Desmopressin (DDAVP) – first line
  ▪ vWF concentrates if non-responsive to DDAVP

Thrombocytopenia

845. What two viral infections must be evaluated for when working up a patient with unexplained thrombocytopenia?
> HIV
> Hepatitis C

846. What are the two most commonly used treatments for patients with idiopathic thrombocytopenia purpura (ITP)?

> IVIg
> Steroids

847. What are the clinical characteristics of heparin induced thrombocytopenia (HIT)?

> Platelet decrease >50% in patients on heparin
> Thromboembolic event 5-10 days after starting heparin

848. What are the components of the **4T** score? What is this score used for?

> **T**hrombocytopenia (percentage decrease and nadir)
> **T**iming of thrombocytopenia
> **T**hrombosis or other sequelae
> **T**hrombocytopenia (other etiologies)
> It can be used to risk stratify for HIT in patients with acute thrombocytopenia and recent heparin exposure

849. What is the gold standard for confirming HIT?

> Serotonin release assay

850. What is the treatment for HIT? When should each be avoided? When should treatment be started?

> Argatroban: Avoid in patients with hepatic dysfunction
> Fondaparinux: Avoid in patients with renal failure
> Start it immediately if clinical suspicion is high
  ▪ Do not wait for confirmatory tests

Transfusion Medicine

851. What is the transfusion threshold for most patients?
> Hemoglobin of ≤ 7

852. What causes an acute hemolytic transfusion reaction?
> ABO incompatibility

853. What causes a delayed hemolytic transfusion reaction?
> Delayed emergence of an alloantibody that causes clearance of transfused blood within 2-10 days

854. What causes a febrile nonhemolytic transfusion reaction? When does this typically occur?
> Donor anti-leukocyte antibodies reacting with recipient leukocytes
> Within 6 hours of transfusion.

Miscellaneous Disorders

Anti-Phospholipid Syndrome (APLS)

855. What blood tests are used to diagnose anti-phospholipid syndrome (APLS)?
> Must test positive to ≥1 of the following:
> - Anticardiolipin (serologic test)
> - Anti B2 glycoprotein (serologic test)
> - Lupus anticoagulant (series of coagulation tests)

856. To be diagnosed with APLS, the patient must have at least one of which three clinical symptoms?

> Vascular thrombosis
> At least 1 fetal death before 34 weeks
> At least 3 spontaneous abortions before 10
  weeks

857. What is the anticoagulant of choice in the long-term management of APLS?

> Warfarin

Hypereosinophilia

858. What are the most common etiologies for hypereosinophilia?

> **N**eoplasm
> **A**llergy/Asthma
> **A**drenal insufficiency
> **C**ollagen vascular disease (EGPA)
> **P**arasite
  - Remember: "**NAACP**"

Paroxysmal Nocturnal Hemoglobinuria (PNH)

859. What hematologic syndrome should be considered on the differential for a patient presenting with unexplained Budd-Chiari Syndrome and hemolysis?

> Paroxysmal nocturnal hemoglobinuria (PNH)

860. On flow cytometry, what cell surface markers are absent in PNH?

> CD55 and CD59

861. What medication reduces hemolysis, hemoglobinuria, and transfusion need in PNH?

> Eculizumab

Felty Syndrome

862. What triad is present in Felty Syndrome?
   ➤ Neutropenia
   ➤ Splenomegaly
   ➤ Rheumatoid arthritis

Myelodysplastic Syndrome (MDS)

863. What abnormalities can be seen on CBC and peripheral smear in patients with MDS?
   ➤ Cytopenia in at least two cell lines
   ➤ Morphologic abnormalities of RBC
   ➤ Pseudo-Pelger-Huet anomaly

864. Why is it important to know if MDS involves the 5q chromosome?
   ➤ Lenalidomide is effective for treating anemia in low risk MDS with 5q deletion

865. What is the treatment for low risk MDS?
   ➤ Observation
   ➤ Supportive transfusion
   ➤ Lenalidomide for patients with a 5q deletion

866. What is the treatment for high risk MDS?
   ➤ Allogeneic HSCT for young, healthy patients
   ➤ Azacytidine or decitabine for patients who are not candidates for HSCT
   ➤ Luspatercept (MEDALIST Trial, 2020)

867. Why are patients with high-risk MDS treated more aggressively?
   ➤ To reduce the risk of progression to AML

Hematologic Oncology

Leukemias

868. A young patient presenting with pancytopenia, coagulopathy, and violaceous nontender cutaneous plaques should be evaluated for what hematologic condition?

➤ Acute myeloid leukemia (AML)

869. What finding on a peripheral blood smear is pathognomonic for AML? What is the translocation?

➤ Auer Rods

➤ t(15:17)

870. What is the treatment of AML (non-APML)?

➤ Cytarabine plus anthracycline (7 + 3)

➤ Older patients treat with hypomethylating agent (ie. decitabine/azacytidine ± venetoclax)

871. What is the treatment in APML?

➤ All-trans retinoic acid (ATRA)

872. What is the syndrome and findings that can classically be associated with ATRA as an adverse effect?

➤ Differentiation syndrome

➤ Fever, pulmonary infiltrates, hypoxemia

873. What is the treatment for differentiation syndrome?

➤ Dexamethasone

874. What is the classic appearance hairy cell leukemia on a peripheral blood smear?

➤ Thread like projections emanating from cell surface (hairy cells)

875. What is the treatment for hairy cell leukemia?

> Cladribine

Lymphomas

876. How is a diagnosis of lymphoma made?

> Excisional biopsy
  - NOT a core biopsy

877. Why is it important to have an excisional biopsy, as opposed to a core biopsy?

> Visualization of the lymph node architecture

878. What are the two main groupings when it comes to classifying lymphomas?

> Hodgkin's and non-Hodgkin's lymphomas

879. What chromosomal translocation is present in follicular lymphoma?

> t(14:18)

880. What are the two classic findings on peripheral blood smear for chronic lymphocytic leukemia (CLL)?

> Lymphocytosis
> Smudge cells

881. Patients with CLL are at risk for what autoimmune hematologic disorders?

> Immune thrombocytopenia (ITP)
> Hemolytic anemia

882. In patients who require treatment for CLL, what is the most commonly used first line medication? What is the most common side effect of this medication?

> Ibrutinib
> Increased bleeding risk and cardiac arrhythmias

883. Where in the world is Burkitt lymphoma endemic? How does it present?

> Equatorial Africa and New Guinea
> Jaw or facial bone tumor

884. What is the classic appearance pathologically in a patient with Burkitt's lymphoma?

> "Starry-sky" pattern

885. What is the classic pathological finding for Hodgkin's lymphoma?

> Reed-Sternberg cells

886. What is the treatment for Hodgkin's lymphoma?

> ABVD (**A**driamycin [doxorubicin/hydroxydaunorubicin], **B**leomycin, **V**inblastine, **D**acarbazine)
  - Followed by radiation therapy

887. For a young woman who had mediastinal Hodgkin's lymphoma that is now cured, what malignancy should she be screened for annually? How should this be evaluated?

> Breast cancer
> MRI

888. What is the most commonly utilized chemotherapy regimen for diffuse large b-cell lymphoma (DLBCL)?

> R-CHOP (**R**ituximab, **C**yclophosphamide, Doxorubicin **H**ydrochloride, Vincristine [**O**ncovin], **P**rednisone)

889. How do T-Cell non-Hodgkin lymphomas (NHL) often present?

> Rash (mycosis fungoidies)

890. What is the treatment for early stage cutaneous T-cell NHL?

 ➢ Topical steroids

891. What cardiac test should be obtained before starting anthracyclines? Why?

 ➢ Echocardiogram

 ➢ Can cause a non-ischemic cardiomyopathy

892. What two chemotherapeutics may cause acute gross hematuria?

 ➢ Cyclophosphamide

 ➢ Ifosfamide

893. What virus is associated with post-transplant lymphoproliferative disease (PTLD)?

 ➢ EBV

Myeloproliferative Neoplasms

894. Chronic myeloid leukemia (CML) is associated with what chromosomal translocation?

 ➢ t(9:22)

 ▪ Philadelphia chromosome

895. What gene is associated with CML?

 ➢ BRC-ABL gene

896. What group of medications can provide long term disease control and induce remission in CML?

 ➢ Tyrosine kinase inhibitors

 ▪ 1st generation: Imatinib

 ▪ 2nd + generation: Dasatinib, nilotinib, bosutinib and other TKIs

897. What mutation is commonly found in patients with myeloproliferative neoplasms?

> $JAK2^{V617F}$

898. In essential thrombocytosis, what is the treatment for low-risk and high-risk patients?

> Low risk: Aspirin
> High risk: Interferon-alpha or hydroxyurea plus aspirin

899. What do you expect to happen to erythropoietin levels in polycythemia vera (PV)?

> Decrease

900. What are the three most common causes of secondary polycythemia?

> Cigarette smoking
> Obstructive sleep apnea
> Hypoxia (ie. congenital heart disease, COPD)

901. What is first line treatment for PV? What is the goal?

> Therapeutic phlebotomy
> HCT <45%

902. What findings on peripheral blood smear are classically seen in primary myelofibrosis?

> Teardrop cell
> Leukoerythroblastosis: Nucleated red cells, circulating blasts

Plasma Cell Dyscrasias

903. What are the five signs and symptoms of multiple myeloma?

> **I**nfection
> hyper**C**alcemia
> **R**enal failure

> <u>A</u>nemia
> <u>B</u>one disease (ie. lytic lesions, fractures)
  - Remember: "<u>I CRAB</u>"

904. What two findings are present in patients with multiple myeloma requiring therapy?

> Bone marrow clonal plasma cells >10% or biopsy proven plasmacytoma
> Myeloma defining events ("I CRAB" criteria)

905. What three biomarkers or radiographic findings are associated with near inevitable progression to end organ damage, and are considered to be equivalent to myeloma defining events?

> ≥60% (<u>S</u>ixty) clonal plasma cells in the marrow
> <u>Li</u>ght chain ratio ≥100
> <u>M</u>RI with more than one focal lesion
  - Together, known as the "<u>SLiM</u>" criteria

906. What are the treatment options for multiple myeloma?

> Proteasome inhibitor (ie. bortezomib)
> Immunomodulatory agents (ie. lenalidomide, pomalidomide, thalidomide)
> Monoclonal antibody to CD38 (ie. daratumumab)
> Steroids
> Alkylating agent (ie. melphalan or cyclophosphamide) if non-transplant candidate
> Auto-HSCT

907. What differentiates smoldering multiple myeloma from multiple myeloma?

> Myeloma defining events ("I CRAB" criteria)

908. What three findings need to be present to be diagnosed with monoclonal gammopathy of unknown significance (MGUS)? What is the treatment?

> Diagnosis:
>   - Serum monoclonal protein <3 g/dL
>   - Bone marrow clonal plasma cells <10%
>   - No end organ damage
> Treatment: Observation

909. What is the hallmark pathologic finding on a biopsy for a patient with AL amyloidosis?

> Apple green birefringence under polarized light with congo red staining

910. What cardiac findings can be seen in AL amyloidosis?

> Low voltage ECG
> Restrictive cardiomyopathy
> Conduction disorders

911. What are the symptoms of hyper-viscosity in Waldenstrom macroglobulinemia?

> Headaches, blurred vision, altered mental status

912. What is the treatment for hyper-viscosity syndrome in Waldenstrom macroglobulinemia?

> Emergent plasmapheresis

7

INFECTIOUS
DISEASE

Microbiology

The Basics

913. What component of the cell wall is unique to gram positive organisms? What color is it on gram stain?

> ➤ Lipoteichoic acid
> ➤ Blue or purple

914. What component of the cell is unique to gram-negative organisms? What color is it on gram stain?

> ➤ Endotoxin/Lipopolysaccharide (LPS)
> ➤ Pink

915. What is the difference between bactericidal and bacteriostatic antibiotics?

> ➤ Bactericidal: Kills the bacteria
> ➤ Bacteriostatic: Prevents further replication of the bacteria

Gram Positive Bacteriology

Staphylococcus

916. What clinically relevant genus of bacteria are gram positive cocci in clusters and catalase positive?

> ➤ Staphylococcus

917. Is Staphylococcus aureus coagulase positive or negative?

> ➤ Coagulase positive

918. What protein is structurally different in methicillin resistant S. aureus (MRSA) as compared to methicillin sensitive S. aureus (MSSA)?

> ➤ Penicillin binding protein

919. What clinical features warrant antibiotic coverage for a S. aureus cellulitis?

> Purulent drainage or abscess

920. In a patient with pneumonia, what test can be done to rule out MRSA as the causative organism?

> MRSA nasal swab

921. What viral pneumonia is S. aureus pneumonia classically associated with as a potential "super-infection"?

> Influenza pneumonia

922. What imaging should be obtained in all patients with S. aureus bacteremia? Why?

> Echocardiogram to evaluate for endocarditis

923. What antibiotics are most effective at treating MSSA?

> Nafcillin, oxacillin, or cefazolin

924. Why is it important to switch to nafcillin, oxacillin, or cefazolin from vancomycin when a patient with S. aureus is confirmed to have MSSA (as opposed to MRSA)?

> These antibiotics are bactericidal
>   ▪ Vancomycin is bacteriostatic
> Vancomycin trough levels can be subtherapeutic, which can impact clinical efficacy

925. What is the most common antibiotic used to treat MRSA infection?

> Vancomycin

926. What is the treatment for "Red-Man syndrome"?

> Decrease the rate of vancomycin infusion
>   ▪ This is not a true allergy

927. In MRSA pneumonia, which anti-MRSA antibiotic should be avoided?

> Daptomycin (does not have activity in the lungs)

928. What types of clinically relevant Staphylococcus are coagulase negative?

> S. epidermidis, S. saprophyticus, S. lugdunensis

929. When is S. epidermidis pathogenic?

> When it infects prosthetic devices or catheters

930. What type of infection does S. saprophyticus most commonly cause?

> Urinary tract infection

Streptococcus

931. What genus of bacteria appears as gram positive cocci in chains that are catalase negative?

> Streptococcus

932. What are the three mechanisms in which Group A Strep (S. pyogenes) can be pathogenic?

> Direct pyogenic infection
> Toxin-mediated
> Immunologic

933. What are the two most common presenting symptoms of Group A Strep (GAS) in adults?

> Pharyngitis
> Skin and soft tissue infection

934. Does Staph or Strep cause the majority of cellulitis infections?

> Strep

935. What are the classic physical exam findings of Scarlet Fever?

➤ Scarlet rash with sandpaper-like texture and a strawberry tongue

936. In Streptococcus mediated glomerulonephritis, approximately how long after the acute Strep infection will the patient develop glomerulonephritis?

➤ 2-3 weeks

937. What toxin-mediated complication of Group A Strep can be rapidly progressive and fatal without emergent surgical debridement or amputation?

➤ Necrotizing fasciitis

938. What are the five major manifestations of acute rheumatic fever?

➤ Polyarthritis (**J**oints)
➤ Carditis (**O** looks like a heart)
➤ Subcutaneous **N**odules
➤ **E**rythema marginatum
➤ **S**ydenham chorea
  ▪ Remember: "**JONES**" criteria

939. How does S. pneumoniae appear on gram stain?

➤ Gram positive diplococci

940. What are the four most common clinical manifestations of S. pneumoniae?

➤ Pneumonia
➤ Meningitis
➤ Otitis Media (especially in children)
➤ Sinusitis

941. What intravenous antibiotic is typically used empirically to treat S. Pneumoniae pneumonia in patients admitted to the hospital?

➤ Ceftriaxone

942. For penicillin-resistant S. pneumoniae meningitis, what antibiotics are used for treatment?

➢ Vancomycin and ceftriaxone

943. In suspected pneumococcal meningitis, other than antibiotics, what other medication should be given concurrently or prior to antibiotics?

➢ Dexamethasone

944. S. viridans colonizes what part of the human body?

➢ Oropharynx

945. What type of infection is S. viridans most commonly associated with?

➢ Endocarditis

946. Group B Strep most commonly causes infections in which patient demographic?

➢ Babies

947. A patient with S. bovis bacteremia should be evaluated for what underlying malignancy?

➢ Colon cancer

Clostridium

948. What food can put babies at risk of getting C. botulinum?

➢ Honey

949. What are two of the biggest risk factors for C. difficile?

➢ Prior antibiotic use
➢ Recent hospitalization or long-term care facility residence

950. What is seen on colonoscopy for patients with severe C. difficile?

> Pseudomembranes

951. What complication should patients with severe C. difficile be monitored closely for?

> Toxic megacolon

952. What is first line treatment for C. difficile?

> Oral vancomycin

953. What invasive procedure is considered curative for patients with recurrent C. difficile?

> Fecal microbiota transplant (FMT)

Listeria

954. What foods are associated with Listeria monocytogenes?

> Unpasteurized dairy products
> Deli meats

955. What clinical illness does listeria cause in immunocompromised adults?

> Meningitis

Actinomyces & Nocardia

956. When distinguishing Actinomyces from Nocardia, which stains weakly acid fast positive?

> Nocardia

957. What antibiotic is used to treat Actinomyces?

> Penicillin

958. What antibiotic is typically included as part of a first-line regimen to treat Nocardia?

> Sulfonamides

Enterococcus

959. What antibiotic is most commonly used to treat vancomycin resistant enterococcus?

> ➢ Linezolid

Gram Negative Bacteriology

Neisseria

960. What is the morphology of the Neisseria genus on gram stain?

> ➢ Gram-negative diplococci

961. What is the method of transmission of N. meningitidis? Which two oral medications can be used for prophylaxis for close contacts of patients diagnosed with N. meningitis? What antibiotic is used for treatment?

> ➢ Transmission: Respiratory and oral secretions
> ➢ Prophylaxis: Rifampin and ciprofloxacin
> ➢ Treatment: Ceftriaxone

962. What is Waterhouse-Friderichsen syndrome?

> ➢ Adrenal infarction that results in adrenal insufficiency in patients with disseminated N. meningitides

963. What type of rash is seen most commonly in meningococcemia?

> ➢ Petechial rash

964. What coinfection must be considered in a patient diagnosed with N. gonorrhoeae?

> ➢ Chlamydia trachomatis

H. influenzae

965. What gram-negative coccobacillus can cause epiglottitis in children?

> Haemophilus influenzae

966. For non-CNS infections of H. influenzae, what antibiotic is used for treatment?

> Amoxicillin-clavulanate

Legionella

967. What gram-negative rod spreads via contaminated water sources and can cause severe pneumonia?

> Legionella pneumophilia

968. What two antibiotic classes can be used to treat legionella?

> Macrolides

> Fluoroquinolones

Pseudomonas

969. Pseudomonas UTI can cause urine to turn which color?

> Green

970. What organism classically causes otitis externa?

> Pseudomonas aeruginosa

▪ Otitis externa can be severe in diabetics

971. What two cephalosporins have activity against pseudomonas?

> Ceftazidime (later 3rd generation)

> Cefepime (4th generation)

E. coli

972. Which E. coli serotype is most commonly associated with hemolytic uremic syndrome (HUS)?
  ➢ O157:H7

973. In a patient with E. coli bacteremia that is ceftriaxone resistant, but piperacillin-tazobactam sensitive, what is the antibiotic class of choice?
  ➢ Carbapenem

974. What pathogen is the most common etiology of a urinary tract infection (UTI)?
  ➢ E. coli

Salmonella

975. What bacteria classically causes diarrhea, salmon-colored macules on abdomen and trunk, and pulse-temperature dissociation?
  ➢ Salmonella typhi

976. Where in the body can salmonella typhi remain latent and result in a carrier state?
  ➢ Gallbladder

977. What household pets are associated with salmonella infection?
  ➢ Reptiles and amphibians

978. What comorbidity is a risk factor for salmonella osteomyelitis?
  ➢ Sickle cell anemia

Campylobacter

979. What are two complications that can be seen after infection with Campylobacter jejuni?

> Guillain Barre Syndrome
> Reactive arthritis

Vibrio

980. Vibrio vulnificus infection can be lethal in patients with what underlying comorbidity?

> Cirrhosis

Yersinia

981. What gram-negative rod causes bloody diarrhea that can mimic appendicitis or Crohn's disease?

> Yersinia enterocolitis

H. pylori

982. What are two reasons it is important to treat Helicobacter pylori?

> It can reduce gastritis and peptic ulcer disease
> It reduces risk for gastric cancer and lymphoma

983. What medications comprise the "triple therapy" needed to treat H. pylori?

> Amoxicillin
> Omeprazole (or any PPI)
> Clarithromycin

984. What are 3 ways to confirm eradication of H. pylori?

> Biopsy
> H. pylori stool antigen
> Urea breath test

Leptospirosis

985. Where in the environment is leptospirosis found? What eye findings are seen in patients with leptospirosis?

> ➤ In fresh water contaminated with animal urine
> ➤ Eye finding: Photophobia with conjunctival suffusion

Lyme Disease

986. Which gram-negative bacteria causes Lyme disease? What is the name and appearance of the characteristic rash associated with Lyme disease?

> ➤ Borrelia burgdorferi
> ➤ Erythema migrans: Bulls-eye morphology

987. What cardiac complication can be seen in Lyme disease?

> ➤ Heart block

988. What is the treatment for uncomplicated Lyme disease? Complicated Lyme disease?

> ➤ Uncomplicated: Doxycycline
> ➤ Complicated (i.e. neurological or cardiac involvement): Ceftriaxone

Syphilis

989. Which gram-negative bacteria causes Syphilis?

> ➤ Treponema pallidum

990. Primary syphilis is characterized by what finding? What symptoms can be present in secondary syphilis? Tertiary syphilis?

> ➤ Primary syphilis:

- Painless chancre
- Secondary syphilis:
  - Maculopapular rash involving palms/soles
  - Condyloma lata
  - Lymphadenopathy
  - Nonspecific constitutional symptoms (ie. fatigue, fevers, arthralgias)
- Tertiary syphilis:
  - Tabes dorsalis
  - Gummas
  - General paresis
  - Aortitis

991. What tests are most commonly used for screening (high sensitivity) and confirmation (high specificity) of Syphilis?
  - Screening: Rapid plasma regain (RPR), Venereal Disease Research Laboratory (VDRL)
  - Confirmation: Fluorescent treponemal antibody absorption (FTA-ABS)

992. What is the treatment for syphilis?
  - Penicillin

993. What is the Jarish-Herxheimer reaction?
  - Flu-like symptoms that can be seen in patients with syphilis after starting penicillin

Rocky Mountain Spotted Fever

994. If a patient was recently in North Carolina and has a fever and rash that starts at the ankles and wrists and progresses to the trunk, including palms and soles, what illness should you consider?

> Rocky Mountain Spotted Fever

995. What organism causes Rocky Mountain Spotted Fever? What is the treatment?

> Organism: Rickettsia rickettsii
> Treatment: Doxycycline

Miscellaneous

996. What organisms can cause pelvic inflammatory disease (PID)?

> Neisseria gonorrhea
> Chlamydia trachomatis

997. What organism causes classic "walking pneumonia" and what antibiotics can be used to treat it?

> Mycoplasma pneumoniae
> Macrolides, fluoroquinolones, or doxycycline

Mycobacteria

998. When evaluating a PPD, what clinical exam finding should be measured when assessing the patient?

> Induration (not erythema)

999. What is considered a positive PPD in a healthy patient? In a healthcare worker, diabetic or dialysis patient? In patients with HIV infection or on immunosuppressive medications?

> Healthy:
  ▪ ≥15 mm of induration
> Healthcare worker, diabetic, or dialysis patient:
  ▪ >10 mm of induration

> Patient with HIV infection or on immunosuppressive medications:
  - ≥5 mm of induration

1000. Other than exposure to tuberculosis, what can cause a PPD to be positive? What screening test should be performed in these individuals?

> BCG vaccination
> Interferon gamma release assay (IGRA aka QuantiFERON gold)

1001. If a patient has a newly positive PPD, what test must be performed to evaluate for active tuberculosis?

> Chest x-ray

1002. Which two medications can be used as part of different regimens to treat latent tuberculosis?

> Isoniazid
> Rifamycin based medications (ie. rifampin or rifapentine)

1003. On chest imaging, which lobe of the lung does pulmonary tuberculosis classically involve?

> Upper lobes

1004. What are the three microbiological methods for diagnosing active pulmonary tuberculosis?

> Sputum AFB Smear
> Molecular testing on sputum (typically nucleic acid amplification)
> Mycobacterial culture of sputum

1005. In tuberculous meningitis, what is the leukocyte differential? Protein level? Glucose level?

> Lymphocytic pleocytosis
> Elevated protein

➢ Decreased glucose

1006. What four antibiotics are used to treat active tuberculosis?

➢ Isoniazid
  ▪ Given with pyridoxine to reduce risk of peripheral neuropathy
➢ Rifampin
➢ Ethambutol
➢ Pyrazinamide

1007. What two organs are most commonly involved in isoniazid toxicity?

➢ Brain/peripheral nervous system
➢ Liver

1008. Which anti-tuberculous medication can cause bodily fluids to turn red or orange?

➢ Rifampin (or other rifamycin containing compounds)

1009. What is the main toxicity to monitor for with ethambutol use?

➢ Optic neuropathy

Viruses

Herpes

1010. Which Herpes virus typically causes temporal lobe encephalitis? Which causes meningitis?

➢ Encephalitis: HSV-1
➢ Meningitis: HSV-2

1011. Which virus causes roseola in children? Which causes Kaposi sarcoma?

➢ HHV-6

> HHV-8

1012. What dermatologic physical exam finding is seen in Kaposi sarcoma?

> Violaceous papular rash

1013. What is the treatment of Kaposi sarcoma if caught early on, prior to metastatic disease?

> Treat the underlying illness (ie. HIV, reduce immune suppression if transplant patient)

1014. What virus can put solid organ transplant patients at increased risk of post-transplant lymphoproliferative disease (PTLD)?

> Epstein-Barr virus (EBV)

1015. In HIV patients, below what CD4 count is a patient typically at risk for CMV retinitis?

> 50

1016. What is first line systemic antiviral medication for CMV?

> Ganciclovir/valganciclovir (can be used with intravitreal antivirals as well)

Rotavirus & Norovirus

1017. What virus is the most common cause of gastroenteritis in children?

> Rotavirus

1018. What virus is classically known for causing outbreaks of gastroenteritis on cruise ships?

> Norovirus

Measles & Mumps

1019. Other than a rash, what are three of the classic symptoms seen in measles infection?

 ➤ Cough
 ➤ Coryza
 ➤ Conjunctivitis

1020. What rare neurological complication can occur a decade or longer after measles infection?

 ➤ Subacute sclerosing pan-encephalitis (SSPE)

1021. What are the most common symptoms of mumps infection?

 ➤ Parotitis
 ➤ Orchitis
 ➤ Meningitis

Influenza

1022. What class of medicine is the mainstay of treatment for influenza?

 ➤ Neuraminidase inhibitors (ie. oseltamivir)

RSV

1023. What virus can classically cause bronchiolitis in children?

 ➤ RSV

Hepatitis

1024. Which hepatitis viruses can cause acute liver failure?

 ➤ Hepatitis A and B

- **NOT** Hepatitis C
  - ➢ Hepatitis E in pregnant women

1025. What is the antibody/antigen profile in a patient with acute HBV?

  - ➢ HbsAg +, HbeAg +, IgM Anti-HBc

1026. What is the antibody profile for a patient in the "window" period of HBV?

  - ➢ Anti-Hbe and IgM Anti-HBc

HIV

1027. What antibody test is used to screen for HIV? What test is used to confirm HIV?

  - ➢ Screen: ELISA
  - ➢ Confirm: Western blot

1028. The newer versions of the ELISA tests also detect what viral antigen?

  - ➢ P24 antigen

1029. What virus causes demyelinating neurological disease in HIV patients with CD4 <200?

  - ➢ JC Virus

1030. What are the three main differential diagnoses for an AIDS patient with a ring-enhancing lesion on bran MRI?

  - ➢ Toxoplasmosis
  - ➢ Primary CNS lymphoma
  - ➢ Brain abscess

1031. At what threshold, for what organism, and what antibiotic are started for prophylaxis in patients with AIDS?

  - ➢ CD4 <200, bactrim prophylaxis for PJP

➢ CD4 ≤100 and positive toxoplasmosis IgG
   serology, bactrim for toxoplasmosis prophylaxis

1032. What drug class makes up the backbone of HIV regimens for treatment-naive patients?

➢ Nucleoside reverse transcriptase inhibitors
   (NRTIs)

1033. What drug class is most commonly used for the third medication for HIV antiretroviral therapy?

➢ Integrase inhibitors (in addition to two NRTIs)

1034. What is immune reconstitution inflammatory syndrome (IRIS)?

➢ Paradoxical worsening of pre-existing infectious
   process after the initiation of antiretroviral
   therapy

1035. What is the treatment for IRIS?

➢ Continue HIV anti-retroviral
➢ Treatment for the underlying opportunistic
   infection
➢ Consider steroids in severe cases

1036. Which two infections in HIV must a clinician consider deferring the initiation of HAART until the underlying infection is treated, due to concerns for possible catastrophic side effects from IRIS?

➢ Cryptococcal meningitis
➢ Tuberculous meningitis

Miscellaneous

1037. What are the TORCH infections? Why are they important?

➢ Toxoplasmosis

> Other (ie. Syphilis, HIV, VZV, Parvovirus B-19)
> Rubella
> CMV
> HSV2
> They can pass from mother to fetus, typically via transplacental transmission, and result in birth defects

1038. What travel associated virus can be characterized by high fevers, rash, and debilitating arthralgias that can last months?

> Chikungunya virus

1039. What travel associated virus can present with non-specific constitutional symptoms, but has been shown to cause birth defects in children of pregnant women?

> Zika virus

1040. What travel associated virus is associated with "break-bone fever", and in rare cases, results in hemorrhagic shock?

> Dengue virus

Fungi

1041. In what part of the United States is histoplasmosis endemic? What outdoor hobby is associated with it?

> Mississippi and Ohio River valley
> Spelunking (cave exploration)

1042. In what part of the United States is blastomycosis endemic? How does it appear under the microscope?

> Southeastern United States (east of Mississippi River)
> Broad based budding yeast

1043. If a patient returns from a trip to Arizona with fevers, arthralgias, and erythematous papules on their shins, what fungal organism should be on your differential?

> Coccidiomycosis

1044. What are the five different forms of pulmonary aspergillus?

> Aspergilloma
> Aspergillus nodule
> Chronic cavitary pulmonary aspergillus, chronic fibrosing pulmonary aspergillosis
> Invasive pulmonary aspergillosis
> Allergic bronchopulmonary aspergillus (ABPA)

1045. What is the treatment for invasive aspergillus?

> Voriconazole

1046. What fungal organism causes thrush?

> Candida

1047. What fungal meningitis are AIDS patients at risk for which often has an elevated opening pressure and requires serial lumbar punctures to reduce ICP?

> Cryptococcal meningitis

1048. What is the initial treatment for cryptococcus meningitis?

> Amphotericin B and flucytosine

1049. What is the typical presentation and imaging pattern of Pneumocystis jirovecii pneumonia (PJP)?

> Dyspnea on exertion, hypoxia, diffuse ground glass opacities on chest imaging

1050. What is the first line treatment and dose for PJP?

> Bactrim 15-20 mg/kg/day (it is the trimethoprim component of Bactrim that treats PJP)

1051. What are the thresholds in which steroids should be given for a patient with PJP pneumonia?

> A-a gradient ≥35
> PaO2 <70
> O_2 sat <92% on room air

1052. What fungal organisms do not contain (1,3)-Beta-D-Glucan (Fungitell test)?

> Cryptococcus
> Rhizopus, mucor, rhizomucor
> Blastomycosis

Parasites

1053. What protozoan infection manifests as foul smelling, fatty diarrhea, and what is the treatment?

> Giardia
> Treatment: Metronidazole

1054. What organism presents as bloody diarrhea and can also cause liver cysts?

> Entamoeba histolytica

1055. In a traveler returning from a tropical region with fevers, what must be evaluated as one of the first infections on the differential?

> Malaria

1056. What are the three preferred malaria treatment regimens for chloroquine resistant malaria?

- ➤ Artesunate (severe malaria)
- ➤ Artemisinin based combination therapy
- ➤ Atovaquone-Proguanil

1057. What parasitic organism can cause dilated cardiomyopathy, megacolon, or megaesophagus?

- ➤ Trypanosoma cruzi (Chagas disease)

1058. In a patient on high dose steroids with a significant increase in their eosinophil count, what parasitic infection must be evaluated for?

- ➤ Strongyloides stercoralis

1059. What parasite, classically seen in sheep herders, can cause liver cysts that should not be aspirated due to risk of anaphylaxis?

- ➤ Echinococcus granulosus

1060. What tapeworm can cause neurocysticercosis?

- ➤ Taenia solium

1061. What organism appears as acid-fast cysts in the stool and can cause watery diarrhea in AIDS patients?

- ➤ Cryptosporidium

1062. What is the treatment for CNS toxoplasmosis in an AIDS patient?

- ➤ Sulfadiazine
- ➤ Pyrimethamine
- ➤ Leucovorin

1063. Which organism has snails as the host and can cause fibrosing liver disease or squamous cell carcinoma of bladder?

- ➤ Schistosomiasis

1064. In the US, what other infections can coexist with Lyme disease transmitted by the deer tick (Ixodes scapularis)?

> Babesiosis
> Human granulocytic anaplasmosis

1065. What hematologic findings is present in babesiosis?

> Hemolysis

1066. What are the two antimicrobial regimens used to treat babesiosis?

> Atovaquone and azithromycin
> Clindamycin and quinine

1067. What hematologic abnormalities are commonly present in anaplasmosis and ehrlichiosis?

> Leukopenia and thrombocytopenia

Miscellaneous

1068. What musculoskeletal injury are fluoroquinolones associated with?

> Tendon rupture

1069. What is the usual cell count profile, glucose, and protein level for bacterial meningitis?

> Neutrophilic pleocytosis
> Low glucose
> High protein

1070. What is the usual cell count profile, protein, and glucose in viral meningitis?

> Lymphocytic pleocytosis
> Elevated protein
> Normal glucose

Infectious Disease

1071. What are the two most common etiologies of bacterial meningitis?
- Streptococcus pneumoniae
- Neisseria meningitidis

1072. Why is a lumbar puncture contraindicated in brain abscess?
- Potential to increase intracranial pressure and cause herniation

1073. In left-sided infective endocarditis, what are the indications for valve surgery?
- Heart block
- Decompensated heart failure
- Paravalvular/aortic abscess
- Persistent infection on appropriate antimicrobial therapy
- Difficult to treat pathogen (ie. multidrug resistant)

1074. What antibiotic regimen is used for empiric treatment of meningitis?
- Ceftriaxone and vancomycin
  - Add ampicillin in patients ≥50 years old

1075. What physical exam findings differentiate bacterial vaginosis (BV), trichomoniasis, and candida vulvovaginitis?
- BV: Thin, white discharge with fishy odor
- Trichomoniasis: Frothy, grey-green foul-smelling discharge
- Candida: Thick, cottage cheese discharge

1076. What is the treatment for BV, trichomoniasis, and candida vulvovaginitis?

- BV: Metronidazole
- Trichomoniasis: Metronidazole
- Candida: Fluconazole

8

NEPHROLOGY

Acute Kidney Injury (AKI)

1077. What is the clinical definition of acute kidney injury (AKI)?

> Within 48 hours: Increase in serum creatinine (Cr) ≥0.3 mg/dL, increase in serum Cr ≥1.5x the baseline, urine output <0.5 mL/kg/hr x 6 hours

1078. What two formulas may be calculated to help differentiate prerenal and acute tubular necrosis (ATN)? What values are indicative of each?

> Fractional excretion of sodium FENa
  - <1% suggestive of prerenal disease
  - >2% suggestive of ATN
> Fractional excretion of urea FEUrea
  - <35% suggestive of prerenal disease
  - >50% suggestive of ATN

1079. Which formula(s) have been shown to be superior in the setting of diuretic use?

> FEUrea
> FE uric acid

1080. What are the common etiologies of post-renal AKI?

> Prostatic etiologies (ie. benign prostatic hyperplasia, prostate cancer), anticholinergic medications, neurogenic bladder, nephrolithiasis, urethral stricture

1081. What are the common causes of intrinsic kidney injury?

> Glomerulonephritis (>15 different forms)
> Vasculitis (ie. anti-glomerular basement membrane antibody disease, ANCA-associated

vasculitis), vascular disease (ie. thrombotic microangiopathy, hemolytic uremic syndrome, scleroderma crisis, disseminated intravascular coagulopathy)

> Acute interstitial nephritis (AIN)
> ATN
> Atheroembolic disease

1082. What are the common causes of prerenal kidney injury?

> Decreased renal perfusion (ie. hypovolemia, CHF, cirrhosis)
> Renal vasoconstriction
  - Typically induced by drugs such as NSAIDs, calcineurin inhibitors
> Diuretic therapy
> ACEi
> ARBs

1083. What are the common causes of AIN?

> Medications (most common)
  - Antibiotics
> Infections, sarcoidosis, Sjogren's syndrome, tubulointerstitial nephritis and uveitis syndrome

1084. What leukocyte cell line has classically been suggested to be present in urine with AIN?

> Eosinophils

1085. What are the common causes of ATN?

> Prolonged pre-renal injury state, septic shock, intra-operative ischemic injury, iodinated contrast nephropathy, rhabdomyolysis

1086. What casts are classically seen under microscopy in ATN?

> Pigmented muddy brown casts

1087. What casts are classically seen in prerenal kidney injury?

> Transparent hyaline casts

1088. What are the most common causes of chronic kidney disease (CKD)? Which is most common?

> Diabetes mellitus (most common)

> Hypertension, genetic (ie. autosomal dominant polycystic kidney disease, Alport syndrome), glomerulonephritis, tubulointerstitial nephritis

Sodium Homeostasis

Regulation

1089. Changes in serum sodium are most likely due to alterations in what?

> Total body water

1090. What are the primary hormone regulators of sodium homeostasis?

> Aldosterone, antidiuretic hormone (ADH), and natriuretic peptides

1091. What hormone is primarily responsible for the regulation of serum sodium concentration via water homeostasis? What are the stimuli for its secretion?

> ADH

> Physiological stimuli: Decreased intravascular volume, hyperosmolality, angiotensin II, thirst

1092. What hormone is the primary regulator of total body sodium? What are the stimuli for its secretion?

> Aldosterone

> Hyperkalemia and hypovolemia

1093. What is the normal value for serum osmolality?

> 280-285 mOsm/kg

1094. What is the normal range for physiological urine osmolality?

> 60-1200 mOsm/L

Hyponatremia

1095. What labs should be obtained in the workup of hyponatremia?

> Urine osmolality, serum osmolality, urine sodium

1096. What are common causes of hypertonic hyponatremia (pseudohyponatremia)?

> Hyperglycemia, hyperlipidemia, hyperproteinemia

1097. What are the common causes of syndrome of inappropriate diuretic hormone (SIADH)?

> Stroke, brain trauma, antipsychotics, antidepressants, cancer, pneumonia, pain, surgery

1098. What are the causes of hypervolemic hypotonic hyponatremia?

> Cirrhosis, congestive heart failure, nephrotic syndrome, renal failure
> ▪ Disorders that lead to a decrease in effective arterial volume

1099. In a patient with acute symptomatic hyponatremia what should be the maximum rate of correction?

> Sodium correction should not exceed 8 mEq/L/d

1100. What could be the fatal adverse event due to overcorrection of serum sodium in a hyponatremic patient?

> Osmotic demyelination syndrome (central pontine myelinolysis)

1101. What is the treatment of SIADH in an asymptomatic patient?

> Free water restriction and treat or remove the underlying cause
> Consider salt tabs if SIADH is chronic

Hypernatremia

1102. What is the most common cause of hypernatremia? Who is this commonly seen in?

> Loss of free water (dehydration)
> Unconscious patients needing tube feeds

1103. What is the treatment of hypernatremia?

> Calculate and replace the free water deficit

1104. How quickly can sodium be corrected? What is the potentially fatal outcome if this is done too quickly in a patient with hyponatremia?

> <0.5 mEq/L/h
> Cerebral edema

Potassium Homeostasis

Hypokalemia

1105. What are the common causes of hypokalemia?

> Insulin, hypothermia, alkalemia, diuretic therapy, GI losses (ie. diarrhea, vomiting), renal losses in polyuria, hyperaldosteronism

1106. What syndromes are associated with hypokalemia due to renal losses of potassium?

> Bartter's syndrome
> Gitelman's syndrome

Hyperkalemia

1107. What are the common causes of hyperkalemia?

> Insulin deficiency, rhabdomyolysis, hemolysis, beta-blockers, acidemia, succinylcholine, AKI, hypoaldosteronism

1108. What are the classic ECG findings of hyperkalemia?

> Peaked T waves
> Increased PR interval
> Widening of the QRS interval
> Loss of P waves
> Sine wave pattern

1109. What are the treatment options for hyperkalemia?

> Kayexalate, patiromer, zirconium cyclosilicate, albuterol, insulin with dextrose, IV calcium gluconate, IV bicarbonate, hemodialysis

1110. What pharmacologic therapy should be administered first in a patient with hyperkalemia and ECG changes?

> IV calcium gluconate

Diuretics

1111. What are the three types of diuretic drug therapies?
> ➢ Thiazides
> ➢ Loop
> ➢ Potassium sparing diuretics

1112. What are the three most commonly used thiazide diuretics? What is their mechanism of action?
> ➢ Chlorthalidone, hydrochlorothiazide, metolazone
> ➢ Inhibit Na-Cl cotransporter in the distal convoluted tubule

1113. What are the three most commonly used loop diuretics? What is their mechanism of action?
> ➢ Bumetanide, furosemide, torsemide
> ➢ Inhibit the Na-K-2Cl transporter in the thick ascending loop of Henle

1114. What are common potassium-sparing diuretics?
> ➢ Spironolactone, eplerenone, triamterene

1115. What are the adverse effects of thiazides? Loop diuretics? Potassium sparing diuretics?
> ➢ Thiazides: Hypomagnesemia, hypokalemia, hyponatremia, and hyperglycemia
> ➢ Loop diuretics: Hypokalemia, ototoxicity, hypersensitivity
> ➢ Potassium sparing diuretics: Hyperkalemia, gynecomastia (spironolactone)

Glomerular Diseases

1116. What are the two typical presentations of glomerulonephritis?

> Nephrotic syndrome: Subacute with heavy proteinuria, hypoalbuminemia, edema and hyperlipidemia
  - Bland urine sediment
  - Proteinuria >3.5 mg/dL
> Nephritic syndrome: Acute with hypertension, elevated creatinine, hematuria and proteinuria
  - Urine microscopy reveals dysmorphic red blood cells or red blood cell casts

1117. What antineutrophil cytoplasmic antibody (ANCA) positive diseases are common causes of glomerulonephritis?

> Eosinophilic granulomatosis with polyangiitis
> Granulomatosis with polyangiitis
> Microscopic polyangiitis

1118. What two organ systems are classically affected by anti-glomerular basement membrane (anti-GBM) disease?

> Kidneys
> Lungs

1119. What are the immune complex-mediated diseases that cause glomerulonephritis?

> Membranoproliferative glomerulonephritis (MPGN)
> IgA nephropathy
> SLE
> Cryoglobulinemia

> Henoch-Schonlein purpura
> Post-infectious glomerulonephritis (PGN)

1120. What are the classic complement patterns (C3, C4) in PGN? IgA nephropathy? MPGN? SLE?

> PGN: Decreased C3
> IgA nephropathy: Normal C3
> MPGN: Decreased C3
> SLE: Decreased C3 and C4

1121. What is the test of choice for suspected glomerulonephritis? What is the most common form of glomerulonephritis?

> Renal biopsy with light microscopy, immunofluorescence and electron microscopy
> IgA nephropathy

1122. What antibody is commonly elevated in patients with PGN?

> Antistreptolysin O antibody (post-streptococcal)

1123. What are the most common glomerular diseases causing nephrotic syndrome?

> Membranous nephropathy
> Minimal change disease
> Focal segmental glomerulosclerosis (FSGS)

1124. What is the most common cause of nephrotic syndrome in adults?

> Idiopathic FSGS

1125. What are the common causes of secondary FSGS?

> HIV
> Drugs (ie. bisphosphonates, NSAIDs)
> Toxins (ie. heroin)

> Obesity
> Reduced nephron mass from pathologic causes

1126. What is the pharmacological treatment of nephrotic syndrome?

> ACEi/ARB
> Treat the underlying disease

Kidney Stones

1127. What mineral component most commonly causes nephrolithiasis?

> Calcium containing stones such as calcium oxalate

1128. What type of stone is a common cause of nephrolithiasis and is radiolucent on x-ray?

> Uric acid-containing stones

1129. What imaging modality is best to evaluate for nephrolithiasis?

> Non-contrast CT

1130. What is the pharmacological therapy for nephrolithiasis? What additional treatment may be used for struvite calculi?

> Alpha-blockers, analgesics, fluid hydration, antibiotics (if a UTI is present)
> Struvite calculi: Urease inhibitors (ie. acetohydroxamic acid)

1131. Stones of what size typically will pass spontaneously? What size are unlikely to pass spontaneously?

> Spontaneously: ≤4 mm in diameter
> Unlikely to pass: ≥10 mm in diameter

1132. What are the indications for urgent urology referral in patients with nephrolithiasis?

> Significant AKI, urosepsis, intractable pain, nausea, or vomiting

1133. What are the primary treatment options for the prevention of uric acid stone recurrence?

> Urine alkalization with K-citrate
> Increase fluid intake >2 L/d
> Decreased uric acid production with a decrease in purine intake
> Xanthine oxidase inhibitors

1134. What are the primary treatment options for the prevention of calcium stone recurrence?

> Increased fluid intake >2 L/d
> Low sodium diet
> Increase food intake rich in potassium
> Maintain daily recommended calcium intake

Acid-Base Homeostasis

1135. What are the common neuromuscular disorders that may lead to respiratory acidosis?

> Amyotrophic lateral sclerosis (ALS), Guillain-Barre, myasthenia gravis

1136. What are two primary pulmonary disorders that may lead to respiratory acidosis?

> COPD
> Asthma

1137. What are common causes of respiratory alkalosis?

> Hyperventilation

- Drugs, pain, anxiety, pulmonary embolism

1138. What are common causes of metabolic acidosis?

> Ingestion (ie. methanol, ethanol, isopropyl alcohol, acetaminophen, salicylates)
> Renal failure
> Ketoacidosis (ie. diabetes, alcoholism, starvation)
> Lactic acidosis

1139. What are renal causes of non-anion gap metabolic acidosis?

> Renal tubular acidosis (RTA)

1140. What are the three main types of RTAs?

> Type I: Defect in the distal tubule hydrogen ion secretion
> Type II: Decreased absorption of bicarbonate in the proximal tubule
> Type IV: Hypoaldosteronism

1141. In what RTA is the serum potassium usually decreased?

> Type I

1142. How can you determine the etiology of metabolic acidosis?

> Check urine chloride to determine whether the alkalosis is saline resistant or responsive
  - Saline resistant: Urine chloride >20 mEq/L
  - Saline responsive: Urine chloride <20 mEq/L

1143. What are the common etiologies of saline resistant metabolic acidosis? Saline responsive metabolic acidosis?

> Saline resistant:
  - Bartter's and Gitelman's syndromes

- Exogenous alkali ingestion
- Hyperaldosteronism
➤ Saline responsive:
  - Laxatives
  - Cystic fibrosis
  - Diuretic use
  - GI losses

9

NEUROLOGY

Headaches

Migraines

1144. What is the most common type of headache in clinical practice?

> ➢ Migraine

1145. What are the characteristics of a migraine headache?

> ➢ **P**ulsatile
> ➢ **O**ne day duration
>> ▪ Typically, range from 4-72 hours
> ➢ **U**nilateral
> ➢ **N**ausea or vomiting
> ➢ **D**isabling
>> ▪ Remember: "**POUND**"

1146. What is first line treatment for a mild to moderate migraine? What treatment may be indicated if there is no response to first line medications?

> ➢ First line: Aspirin, NSAIDs, or tylenol
> ➢ Triptan

1147. In which patients are triptans contraindicated?

> ➢ Patients with coronary artery disease or cerebrovascular disease
> ➢ Brainstem aura (relative contraindication)
> ➢ Hemiplegic migraine (relative contraindication)

1148. In women who have migraines with aura, which medication should be avoided?

> ➢ Estrogen-containing contraceptives

1149. What medications can be considered for migraine prophylaxis?

- ➤ Tricyclic antidepressants
- ➤ Beta blockers
- ➤ Valproic acid
- ➤ Topiramate
- ➤ Venlafaxine
- ➤ Botox
- ➤ Calcitonin gene-related peptide receptor (CGRP) antagonists
  - ▪ Newer medication, but strong data to support utility in migraine prophylaxis

Cluster Headaches

1150. What are the classic characteristics of a cluster headache?
- ➤ Severe unilateral or periorbital headache lasting minutes to hours
- ➤ Unilateral tearing, nasal congestion, or rhinorrhea
- ➤ Ptosis or miosis

1151. What is the treatment for acute cluster headaches? What can be used for prophylaxis?
- ➤ Acute treatment: Triptan (typically subcutaneous or intranasal) or oxygen
- ➤ Prophylaxis: Verapamil

Other Headaches

1152. Which diagnosis should be considered in a patient endorsing severe, unilateral pain on the cheek that is triggered by light touch?
- ➤ Trigeminal neuralgia

1153. A complaint of the "worst headache of their life" should be concerning for which diagnosis?

> Subarachnoid hemorrhage

1154. What is most likely diagnosis in a young, obese woman who complains of headaches and is found to have papilledema on exam? What is the treatment?

> Idiopathic intracranial hypertension (pseudotumor cerebri)

> Treatment: Acetazolamide and weight loss

Seizure Disorders

1155. What is the definition of convulsive status epilepticus?

> Convulsions for ≥5 minutes or at least 2 discrete seizures with incomplete recovery of consciousness between them

1156. For an acute seizure, what medication class is most commonly utilized first?

> Benzodiazepines

1157. For a patient with status epilepticus not previously on anti-epileptic drugs, what medication should be considered after benzodiazepines?

> Phenytoin, valproate, or levetiracetam

  ▪ ESETT trial demonstrated no difference in rate of seizure cessation comparing these three medications

Stroke & Intracerebral Hemorrhage

1158. What are the 5 causative mechanisms in ischemic stroke? What is a widely used classification scheme of ischemia stroke subtypes?

> - Large artery atherosclerosis
> - Cardioembolic
> - Small vessel occlusion
> - Stroke of other determined etiology (ie. carotid dissection, endocarditis, hypercoagulability)
> - Stroke of undetermined etiology (ie. cryptogenic)
> - Classification: TOAST criteria

1159. How does a transient ischemic attack (TIA) differ from a stroke?

> - Tissue based: Symptoms consistent with focal cerebral dysfunction due to a vascular cause without evidence of infarction on neuroimaging
> - Time based: Symptoms consistent with focal cerebral dysfunction due to a vascular cause that last <24 hours

1160. What tests should be done in all patients with a TIA or stroke?

> - CT head without contrast
> - ECG and telemetry
> - Cerebrovascular imaging (head and neck vessels)
> - Echocardiogram
> - Hemoglobin A1c and lipid panel

1161. What risk stratification system can be utilized to decide whether to admit a patient with a TIA?

> - **ABCD²** score of ≥3
>   - **A**ge >60 years

- **B**lood pressure >140/90
- **C**linical symptoms (ie. focal weakness with TIA or speech impairment without weakness)
- **D**uration (more or less than 1 hour)
- **D**iabetes

1162. What is the time window for administration of tissue plasminogen activator (tPA) for ischemic strokes?

> ➤ 4.5 hours

1163. What are the exclusion criteria for tPA administration?

> ➤ Absolute contraindications:
> - Intracranial or systemic hemorrhage
> - SBP >185 or DBP >110 mmHg
> ➤ Relative contraindications:
> - Current use of anticoagulation
> - Increased risk of bleeding (ie. recent ischemic stroke, significant GI bleeding history, coagulopathic)

1164. What imaging is used to diagnose subarachnoid hemorrhage (SAH) in ≥90% of cases?

> ➤ CT head without contrast

1165. If the CT scan is negative, but clinical suspicion is high for SAH, what is the best next test? What would confirm the diagnosis of SAH?

> ➤ Lumbar puncture
> ➤ Xanthochromia

1166. What is the blood pressure goal after subarachnoid hemorrhage to prevent rebleeding?

> ➤ SBP <140 mmHg

1167. What medication should be used after SAH to prevent vasospasm? For how long should it be prescribed?

> Oral nimodipine
> 3 weeks

1168. What is the most common risk factor for intracerebral hemorrhage?

> Hypertension

1169. What are the medications of choice to lower blood pressure in neurological emergencies?

> IV nicardipine
> IV labetalol

1170. Who is at risk for subdural hematomas, even in the absence of trauma?

> Elderly patients
> Patients on anticoagulation
> Alcoholics

Memory Disorders

Dementia

1171. What score on the mini mental exam is consistent with dementia?

> ≤24
  - 20-24: Mild
  - 13-20: Moderate
  - <13: Severe

1172. What should elderly patients with increasing memory loss and decreased functional status be screened for?

> Depression

> Vitamin B12 deficiency
> Hypothyroidism
> Tertiary syphilis

1173. What form of dementia is characterized by mild Parkinsonism and visual hallucinations?

> Dementia with Lewy bodies

1174. What form of dementia is characterized by early and prominent behavioral changes?

> Frontotemporal dementia

Normal Pressure Hydrocephalus

1175. What is the classic triad seen in patients with normal pressure hydrocephalus (NPH)?

> Cognitive impairment
> Gait dysfunction
> Urinary incontinence

Alzheimer's Disease

1176. What are the pharmacologic treatments for Alzheimer's disease?

> Mild to moderate disease: Acetylcholinesterase inhibitors
> Moderate to severe disease: Memantine
>   - Usually in addition to acetylcholinesterase inhibitors, unless they are not well tolerated

Delirium

1177. What is the treatment for delirium?

> Reorientation

➤ Elimination of precipitating factors
➤ Antipsychotics
  ▪ Only used for hyperactive delirium when safety is a concern

Movement Disorders

Parkinson's Disease

1178. What are the classic symptoms of Parkinson's disease?

➤ **T**remor
➤ **R**igidity
➤ **A**kinesia/bradykinesia
➤ **P**ostural instability
➤ **S**huffling gait
  ▪ Remember: "**TRAPS**"

1179. If dementia is present within the first year of Parkinson's symptoms, what diagnosis should be considered?

➤ Dementia with Lewy bodies

1180. What is first line medication for Parkinson's disease?

➤ Levodopa combined with carbidopa

Parkinson Plus Syndromes

1181. What diagnosis should be considered in a patient with Parkinsonism symptoms not responsive to medications and a vertical gaze palsy?

➤ Progressive supranuclear palsy

Demyelinating Disorders

1182. What is required to make the diagnosis of multiple sclerosis (MS)?

- ➢ Dissemination of CNS lesions in space to different parts of the central nervous system (clinically or radiographically)
- ➢ Dissemination of CNS lesions in time (clinically or radiographically)

1183. What is the treatment for a MS flare?

- ➢ IV steroids
  - ▪ As long as there is no underlying infection

1184. Other than MS, what diagnosis should be considered in a patient presenting with optic neuritis?

- ➢ Neuromyelitis optica (NMO)

Amyotrophic Lateral Sclerosis (ALS)

1185. What are the characteristic findings on neurological exam for ALS?

- ➢ Both upper and lower motor neuron involvement

1186. What medication is approved for ALS, but only improves survival by ~3 months?

- ➢ Riluzole

Myasthenia Gravis & Lambert-Eaton Syndromes

1187. What is the pathophysiology of myasthenia gravis?

➢ Autoantibodies against the postsynaptic nicotinic acetylcholine receptor

1188. What antibiotics (2 classes), cardiac medications (2 classes) and electrolyte can be precipitant of myasthenic crisis?

➢ Antibiotics: Aminoglycosides and quinolones
➢ Cardiac medications: Beta blockers and calcium channel blockers
➢ Electrolyte: Magnesium

1189. How does Lambert-Eaton syndrome differ clinically from myasthenia?

➢ Progressive proximal muscle weakness that improves with repetitive movement of affected muscles
  ▪ Opposite of myasthenia which fatigues with time

1190. Which treatment may provide symptomatic relief for mild myasthenia gravis?

➢ Pyridostigmine
  ▪ Provides symptomatic relief but is not disease modifying

1191. What treatment is required for chronic moderate to severe myasthenia gravis?

➢ Immunosuppressive therapy (ie. steroids, mycophenolate, azathioprine, rituximab)

1192. What is the treatment for myasthenic crisis?

➢ Plasmapheresis
➢ IVIG

1193. What should patients with myasthenia be screened for?

> Thymoma

Bell's Palsy

1194. What is the pattern of weakness in a lower motor neuron lesion such as Bell's palsy?

> Weakness of both the upper and lower part of the face (ie. inability to furrow brow, difficulty closing eye, unable to smile or puff out cheeks)

1195. What is the usual presentation for Bell's palsy? What is the treatment?

> Presentation: Unilateral facial weakness in a lower motor neuron distribution
> Treatment: Prednisone, if within 72 hours of onset

Miscellaneous

1196. What are the three most common malignancies that metastasize to the brain?

> Breast
> Lung
> Melanoma

1197. What are the typical features of serotonin syndrome?

> Abrupt onset
> Hyperthermia and autonomic instability
> Tremor
> Hyperreflexia and clonus

1198. What are the typical features of neuroleptic malignant syndrome?

➢ Subacute presentation following use of
  neuroleptic medications
➢ Rigidity with hyporeflexia
➢ Hyperthermia
➢ Altered mental status

Neurology

10

ONCOLOGY

Breast Cancer

1199. What imaging modality may be needed in patients with dense breast tissue?

> Ultrasound

1200. What are the two most important prognostic factors in breast cancer?

> Tumor size
> Axillary lymph node status

1201. What adjuvant systemic therapy is used in premenopausal women with hormone receptor positive non-metastatic breast cancer? What malignancy does this medication increase the risk of?

> Tamoxifen
> Endometrial cancer

1202. What adjuvant systemic therapy is used in postmenopausal women with hormone receptor positive non-metastatic breast cancer?

> Aromatase inhibitors (ie. anastrozole, letrozole, exemestane)

1203. For patients with HER2 positive breast cancer, what two agents are used as adjuvant therapy, in addition to chemotherapy?

> Trastuzumab
> Pertuzumab

1204. What organ should be considered the primary site in a 50 year old woman who is noted to have weight loss, an enlarged, firm, nonmobile axillary lymph node that shows adenocarcinoma on histology, and a mammogram and a PET scan that are negative?

> Breast

Lung Cancer

1205. Horner's Syndrome is concerning for which cancer? What is the classic triad in Horner's Syndrome?

> Lung

> Triad: Ptosis, miosis, and anhidrosis

1206. What hormones are classically secreted by small cell lung cancer (SCLC)?

> ADH

> ACTH

1207. What metabolic abnormality is classically seen in squamous cell carcinoma of the lung? What is the mechanism?

> Hypercalcemia

> Mechanism: PTHrP

1208. What mutation should be present to have a lung cancer patient benefit from erlotinib, gefitinib, or afatinib?

> EGFR mutation

1209. Which lung cancer patients are candidates for surgical resection?

> Stage I or Stage II non-small cell lung cancer (NSCLC)
>
>> ▪ More advanced NSCLC and SCLC are not treated surgically and require chemotherapy +/- radiation

Gastrointestinal Malignancies

1210. What is a known risk factor for gastric cancer and MALT lymphoma?

Oncology

> H. Pylori infection

1211. For localized gastric cancer, what is the treatment?

> Neoadjuvant chemotherapy +/- radiation, followed by surgery

1212. What is the recommended age and interval for an average risk adult for colorectal cancer colonoscopy screening?

> Starting at age 45 through age 75
  - Colonoscopy every 10 years if no adenomas are found

1213. What is the treatment for a patient with familial adenomatous polyposis (FAP)?

> Prophylactic colectomy

1214. What FAP syndrome is also associated with osteomas, thyroid cancers, medulloblastomas, and duodenal ampullary tumors?

> Gardner's Syndrome

1215. Other than colon cancer, what other malignancy is commonly seen in Lynch syndrome?

> Endometrial cancer

1216. What are the diagnostic criteria for hereditary nonpolyposis colon cancers?

> ≥3 relatives with colorectal cancer
  - One relative must be first degree of the other two
> At least 2 successive generations
> One cancer diagnosed before the age 50 years

1217. How does fecal immunochemical test (FIT) differ from Cologuard for colon cancer screening?

> FIT: Directly measures hemoglobin in the stool
> Cologuard: FIT + multitarget stool DNA testing that looks for DNA shed into stool by colon cancers

1218. What is the treatment for Stage I and Stage II colon cancer? What is the treatment for colon cancer with regional lymph node involvement? With one metastatic lesion in the liver?

> Stage I and II: Resection
> Regional lymph node involvement: Resection followed by adjuvant chemotherapy
> Metastatic lesion in the liver: Resection of primary tumor as well as liver lesion

1219. What is the treatment for Stage II and III rectal cancer?

> Combination chemoradiation before surgery with adjuvant chemotherapy after surgery

1220. What tumor marker can be followed in colorectal cancer to monitor response to treatment?

> CEA

1221. What infection is associated with most anal cancers?

> HPV

1222. What is treatment for anal cancer?

> Radiation with concurrent chemotherapy (NOT surgery)

1223. How often and with what modality should patients with cirrhosis be screened for hepatocellular carcinoma (HCC)?

> Every 6 months with ultrasound (some clinicians will alternate ultrasound and MRI)

1224. How is HCC diagnosed?

> On imaging
  - Biopsy is NOT necessary due to characteristics imaging findings

1225. What are the Milan criteria?

> One tumor <5 cm, or 3 tumors <3 cm

1226. What is the significance of the Milan Criteria in HCC?

> If these criteria are met, patient is a candidate for curative liver transplant

1227. What systemic therapy can be used in patients with advanced HCC who are not surgical candidates?

> Sorafenib

1228. Hepatic adenomas are associated with what medication?

> Oral contraceptives

1229. What is the biggest known risk factor for cholangiocarcinoma?

> Primary sclerosing cholangitis (PSC)

1230. Painless jaundice is classically associated with what malignancy?

> Pancreatic cancer

1231. What would be the next step in a patient who presents with painless jaundice and is found to have a pancreas head mass with no distant metastases or vessel involvement?

> Surgical resection with Whipple surgery

Renal & Genitourinary Cancers

1232. What is the next step in management of a 55 year old woman who presents with abdominal bloating and is found to have an adnexal mass with no ascites or metastatic disease?

> ➤ Removal of mass (without biopsy)

1233. Other than BPH or prostate cancer, what can cause PSA to increase?

> ➤ Acute urinary retention
> ➤ Prostatitis

1234. What is the recommended treatment for men with very low risk prostate cancer and life expectancy >10 years?

> ➤ Active surveillance

1235. What congenital abnormality is a risk factor for testicular cancer?

> ➤ Cryptorchidism

1236. What hormone levels should be checked in a testicular mass? What is the next step in a patient who is found to have a solid testicular mass on ultrasonography?

> ➤ Hormones:
>   ▪ AFP
>   ▪ LDH
>   ▪ B-hCG
> ➤ Next step: Inguinal orchiectomy

1237. How is renal cell carcinoma (RCC) usually diagnosed? What hormone does RCC classically produce as part of a paraneoplastic syndrome?

> Diagnosis: CT scan (biopsy is usually avoided because it carries risk of hemorrhage and seeding of malignancy)
> Hormone: EPO

Thyroid Cancer

1238. What is the most common type of thyroid cancer?

> Papillary

1239. What hereditary syndrome is associated with medullary thyroid cancer?

> MEN 2A or 2B

1240. What are the classic findings in MEN 2A and 2B?

> MEN 2A: Medullary thyroid cancer, hyperparathyroidism, pheochromocytoma
> MEN 2B: Medullary thyroid cancer, pheochromocytoma, marfanoid habitus and ganglioneuromas

1241. What diagnostic study should be done for thyroid nodules >1 cm?

> Fine needle aspiration

1242. What is the treatment for papillary and follicular thyroid cancer?

> Thyroidectomy followed by radioiodine therapy
  ▪ Radioiodine therapy not recommended in medullary thyroid cancer because it is not taken up by C cells

Oncologic Emergencies

1243. How is fever defined in neutropenic patients? What is the empiric treatment?

> ➤ Definition:
>> ▪ Single oral temperature >38.3°C
>> ▪ Temperature >38°C sustained for 1 hour
> ➤ Treatment:
>> ▪ Anti-pseudomonal beta lactam agent (ie. cefepime, piperacillin-tazobactam, meropenem)
>> ▪ Vancomycin if evidence of skin and soft tissue infection, catheter related or intravenous line infections

1244. What diagnosis should be considered in a patient with neutropenia and abdominal pain?

> ➤ Typhlitis

1245. When should granulocyte colony stimulating factor (GCSF) be used?

> ➤ When neutropenia associated with chemotherapy is complicated by severe infection with sepsis

1246. What electrolyte abnormalities are seen in tumor lysis syndrome (TLS)? What is the cornerstone of treatment for TLS?

> ➤ Hyperkalemia
> ➤ Hyperuricemia
> ➤ Hyperphosphatemia
> ➤ Hypocalcemia
> ➤ Treatment: Aggressive IV Hydration

1247. What two medications are used for hyperuricemia in TLS if a patient has renal failure?

- ➢ Rasburicase
- ➢ Allopurinol

1248. Above what WBC count should leukocytosis become a concern?

- ➢ Above 50,000 WBC
  - ▪ More common in blast processes, as opposed to CML

1249. What is the treatment for a patient with metastatic cancer presenting with calcium level of 17 mg/dL?

- ➢ Aggressive IV normal saline, can consider using diuretics to augment
- ➢ Bisphosphonate
- ➢ Calcitonin

1250. A patient with lung cancer presents with nausea and vomiting, what is the first imaging study to obtain?

- ➢ CT Head to evaluate for brain metastases

1251. What are the characteristic clinical findings of spinal cord compression? What is the treatment:

- ➢ Clinical findings:
  - ▪ Back pain
  - ▪ Lower extremity weakness
  - ▪ Bowel/bladder dysfunction
  - ▪ Perineal anesthesia
- ➢ Treatment:
  - ▪ IV steroids
  - ▪ Radiation
  - ▪ Emergent surgical decompression followed by emergent surgical decompression

1252. What syndrome should be considered in a patient with a 50-pack year history who presents with facial edema, plethora, swollen right arm and dyspnea?

> SVC Syndrome

Oncology

11

PULMONOLOGY

Pulmonary Physiology

1253. What are the functions of pulmonary surfactant?
> - Decrease alveolar surface tension
> - Prevent alveolar collapse

1254. What are the four measurements of lung volumes?
> - Tidal volume (TV): Air that enters the lungs with each normal effort inspiration
> - Residual volume (RV): Air remaining in lung after maximal expiration
> - Expiratory reserve volume (ERV): Air that can be further exhaled after normal tidal volume expiration
> - Inspiratory reserve volume (IRV): Air that can be inhaled after normal tidal volume inspiration

1255. What are the four capacities measured in the lung?
> - Inspiratory capacity = IRV + TV
> - Functional residual capacity = RV + ERV
> - Vital capacity = TV + IRV + ERV
> - Total lung capacity = IRV + TV + ERV + RV

1256. What is minute ventilation?
> - Total volume of gas entering lungs per minute
>   - Normal is 6-8L/min

1257. What is lung compliance?
> - The amount of pressure required to change lung volume

1258. What shifts the oxygen dissociation curve to the **RIGHT**, causing a decreased affinity of hemoglobin for oxygen, which in turn facilitates unloading of oxygen to tissues?

> $\underline{C}O_2$
> $\underline{A}$ltitude/$\underline{A}$cid
> 2,3-$\underline{D}$PG
> $\underline{E}$xercise
> $\underline{T}$emperature
    - Remember: "**CADET** face **RIGHT**"

1259. How is the pulmonary circulation different from systemic circulation?

> Hypoxic vasoconstriction: A decrease in alveolar oxygen content results in vasoconstriction, shunting blood to areas of the lung with better oxygenation

1260. What is the difference between perfusion and diffusion limited gas exchange?

> Perfusion limited: Gas equilibrates quickly, only way to increase gas exchange is to increase blood flow (ie. CO_2, oxygen in normal lungs)
> Diffusion limited: Gas does not equilibrate by the time blood reaches end of the capillary (ie. CO, Oxygen in emphysema)

1261. What are the five etiologies of hypoxemia? How is the A-a gradient influenced?

> High altitude (normal A-a gradient)
> Hypoventilation (normal A-a gradient)
> V/Q mismatch (increased A-a gradient)
> Decreased DLCO (increased A-a gradient)
> Right to left shut (increased A-a gradient)

1262. Is V/Q mismatch greater in the base or apex of the lung?

> Apex

Pulmonary Infections

1263. A patient with a new upper lobe cavitary lung lesion being admitted to the hospital should be placed on what isolation precautions?

> Airborne isolation until 3 sputum samples are negative for AFBs

1264. What medication resulted in lower 28-day mortality for COVID-19 patients receiving invasive mechanical ventilation or oxygen therapy?

> Dexamethasone

1265. What are the two standard antibiotics and dose for legionella pneumonia?

> Azithromycin 500 mg daily
> Levofloxacin 750 mg daily

1266. At what age should a patient with diabetes, heart, lung, or liver disease get the PPSV23 and PCV13 vaccines?

> One dose of PPSV23 between ages 19-64 years
> PCV13 at age ≥65 years (at least one year after PPSV23)
> Second dose of PPSV23 after age 65 (at least one year after PCV13)

1267. What underlying pulmonary condition is associated with Burkholderia pneumonia?

> Cystic fibrosis

1268. Other than antibiotics and supportive care, what else should be done in an elderly patient who presents with fevers, cough, and dyspnea, and is found to have a right lower lobe pneumonia with a moderate parapneumonic effusion on chest x-ray.?

> Thoracentesis to evaluate for empyema

1269. In a patient with HIV/AIDS and acute pneumothorax, what underlying infection must be considered?

> Pneumocystis jirovecii pneumonia

Obstructive Airway Disease

1270. In COPD, what is the hallmark finding on PFTs?

> A decreased FEV1/FVC ratio of <0.7

1271. What are the characteristic symptoms of chronic bronchitis?

> "Blue Bloater": Productive cough for several months per year for at least 2 years

1272. Via what mechanism does hypoxemia occur in emphysema?

> Reduced DLCO from destruction of alveolar walls

1273. What are the 3 cardinal features of a COPD exacerbation?

> Increase in frequency of severity of cough
> Increase in sputum production or change in caliber
> Increased dyspnea

1274. For COPD patients with at least one hospitalization, what maintenance medications should they be receiving?

> At least two of the following:
> - Long-acting beta 2 agonist (LABA)
> - Long-acting muscarinic agonist (LAMA)
> - Inhaled corticosteroid (ICS)
> - Note: a recent publication in NEJM suggests triple therapy may be superior in reducing exacerbations

1275. What is the first blood test that should be obtained in a patient who presents with a COPD exacerbation and is somnolent? Why?

> ABG to assess for hypercarbic respiratory failure

1276. For a patient with severe chronic bronchitis with recurrent exacerbations requiring oral steroids despite ICS, LABA and LAMA use, what can be added and has been shown to reduce risk of exacerbation and improve lung function?

> Roflumilast

1277. For patients with severe COPD and continued exacerbations despite ICS, LABA and LAMA, what additional oral medication class has been shown to reduce frequency of COPD exacerbations?

> Macrolides

1278. What hereditary disorder can cause panacinar emphysema?

> Alpha 1 antitrypsin deficiency

1279. What are the indications for continuous long-term oxygen therapy for patients with COPD?

> PaO2 ≤55 mmHg

> SpO2 ≤88% on room air at rest

1280. What is the diagnosis in a patient with severe COPD and a dilated right ventricle with reduced function?

> Cor pulmonale

1281. What is the gold standard for asthma diagnosis?

> Methacholine challenge

1282. What is the pathophysiology behind asthma exacerbations?

> Bronchial hyperresponsiveness to a trigger (ie. URI, allergen) which results in reversible bronchoconstriction

1283. What is first line treatment for intermittent asthma

> Albuterol inhaler as needed (short acting bronchodilator – SABA)

1284. What maintenance medication should be used in mild persistent asthma?

> Daily low dose ICS

1285. For a patient admitted with a severe asthma exacerbation, what medications should be administered?

> Albuterol nebulizer

> IV Magnesium

> Systemic steroids

1286. For a patient with persistent refractory asthma despite multiple courses of oral steroids, with an elevated IgE level, what treatment can be considered?

> Omalizumab

1287. For a patient with persistent refractory asthma despite multiple courses of oral steroids, with an elevated eosinophil level, what treatment can be considered?

➢ Mepolizumab

1288. What asthma medication is a leukotriene antagonist?

➢ Montelukast

1289. What medication allergy can be associated with asthma? What nasal finding can be associated asthma?

➢ Aspirin
➢ Nasal polyps

1290. What test can be done in the office, or even at home, and be compared to prior values, to inform you of the severity of an asthma exacerbation?

➢ Peak flow meter

1291. What is the recommended treatment for occasional, exercise induced asthma?

➢ SABA 15-30 minutes before exercise

1292. What should be considered in a patient who presents to the ER with a severe asthma exacerbation and a normal PCO2 on arterial blood?

➢ Impending respiratory failure as they may be tiring out and require intubation

1293. Does a normal in-office spirometry rule out asthma?

➢ No

1294. On PFTs, what defines reversible airway obstruction in response to bronchodilator therapy?

> >12% increase in FEV1 or FVC with a 200 mL
> increase from baseline in either parameter

1295. What are the pulmonary findings in lymphangioleimyomatosis (LAM)? What demographic does it affect?

> Diffuse pulmonary cysts, pneumothoraces, chylous pleural effusions, and obstructive airway disease
> Young women

Restrictive Lung Disease

1296. In restrictive lung disease, what are the characteristic findings on PFTs?

> FEV1/FVC >0.8
> FEV1 and FVC are both reduced, as is total lung capacity

1297. What threshold for total lung capacity is indicative of restrictive lung disease?

> ≤80%

1298. What medications have been shown to slow progression of disease in idiopathic pulmonary fibrosis?

> Nintedanib
> Pirfenidone

1299. What are three diagnostic tests for cystic fibrosis?

> Sweat chloride test
> Nasal potential difference testing
> Genetic CFTR mutation testing

1300. What is treatment for cryptogenic organizing pneumonia (COP)?

> Systemic steroids

1301. What is the best treatment for hypersensitivity pneumonitis?

> ➤ Remove the offending agent

1302. What is the treatment for an asymptomatic patient found to have incidental bilateral hilar lymphadenopathy, suggestive of pulmonary sarcoid, with a normal physical exam and lab values?

> ➤ Observation

1303. Who should be treated for pulmonary sarcoid? What is the treatment? What is seen on sarcoid biopsy?

> ➤ Patients with clinical symptoms from organ dysfunction
> ➤ Steroids
> ➤ Biopsy: Noncaseating granulomas
> ▪ Need to rule out infectious etiology

1304. What are the four hallmarks of Lofgren syndrome?

> ➤ Fever
> ➤ Bilateral hilar lymphadenopathy
> ➤ Erythema nodosum
> ➤ Ankle arthritis

1305. On routine labs, what lab abnormality may be seen in patients with sarcoidosis? Why does this occur?

> ➤ Hypercalcemia
> ➤ Granulomas increase levels of 1 alpha hydroxylase, which increases 1,25 dihydroxy Vitamin D3 and subsequent calcium absorption

1306. What ocular diagnosis is associated with sarcoidosis?

> ➤ Anterior uveitis

1307. In a patient with cystic fibrosis and acute abdominal pain, what diagnosis should you consider?

> Intussusception

1308. What anti-arrhythmic drug classically causes intrinsic pulmonary disease as an adverse effect?

> Amiodarone

1309. What is the only treatment that can improve mortality in idiopathic pulmonary fibrosis?

> Lung transplantation

Pulmonary Hypertension

1310. What are the five groups of pulmonary hypertension (PH)?

> WHO I: Disease localized to small pulmonary arterioles (PAH)
> WHO II: Left heart failure
> WHO III: Intrinsic lung disease
> WHO IV: Chronic thromboembolic pulmonary hypertension (CTEPH)
> WHO V: Miscellaneous

1311. At what mean pulmonary arterial pressure is a patient considered to have pulmonary hypertension?

> 25 mmHg

1312. Other than PAH, what other etiologies can cause WHO I pulmonary hypertension?

> HIV
> Portopulmonary hypertension
> Scleroderma and other connective tissue disorders

1313. How is CTEPH diagnosed?

➤ V/Q scan

1314. What oral medication class can be used for a patient with WHO I PH that responds to nitric oxide?

➤ Calcium channel blockers

1315. Is the pulmonary capillary wedge pressure elevated or decreased in WHO II pulmonary hypertension?

➤ Elevated (typically >12-15)

1316. What is the definitive treatment for chronic thromboembolic pulmonary hypertension?

➤ Pulmonary thromboendoarterectomy

Pleural Disease

1317. In a tension pneumothorax, is the trachea deviated towards or away from the side of the pneumothorax?

➤ Away from side of pneumothorax

1318. What are Lights Criteria?

➤ Pleural fluid protein >0.5 serum protein
➤ Pleural fluid LDH >0.6 serum LDH
➤ Pleural fluid LDH >2/3 upper limits of the laboratory reference range of serum LDH
➤ If any of the above 3 are positive, it is suggestive of an exudative effusion

1319. What are the lab characteristics of a complicated pleural effusion?

➤ pH <7.2
➤ Glucose <60
➤ LDH >3x upper limit of normal in serum

1320. What is the treatment for a complicated pleural effusion?

> Antibiotics
> Chest tube (they are at high risk for developing empyema)

1321. In patients with empyema, other than chest tube and antibiotics, what has been shown to reduce rates of surgical referral and length of hospital stay?

> Instillation of intrapleural tPA and intrapleural deoxyribonuclease via chest tube

1322. In a pleural effusion with >80% lymphocytes, what four diagnoses should be at the top of your differential?

> TB
> Lymphoma
> Rheumatoid arthritis associated pleuritis
> Sarcoid

1323. What pleural fluid study should be sent in a patient with suspected TB associated pleural effusion?

> Adenosine deaminase

1324. What treatment should be considered in a tall, thin man with Marfan Syndrome who presents with acute onset dyspnea, tachycardia, and hypotension with no breath sounds on the right side?

> Needle decompression for tension pneumothorax

1325. When performing a thoracentesis, should you go right above or below the rib with the needle?

> Above the rib (remember the neurovascular bundle runs beneath the ribs)

1326. What is the most common cause of secondary pneumothorax?

> Emphysema

1327. What should be done prior to discharge in a patient with emphysema who had a chest tube placed secondary spontaneous pneumothorax?

> Pleurodesis should be done after the first episode of secondary spontaneous pneumothorax because the risk of recurrence in these patients is up to 50%

1328. In primary spontaneous pneumothorax, after how many occurrences should pleurodesis be pursued?

> Two

Occupational Exposures

1329. Asbestos exposure increases the of which malignancy? Silicosis exposure?

> Asbestos exposure: Mesothelioma
> Silicosis exposure: Tuberculosis

1330. What workplace exposure can cause a sarcoid-like clinical syndrome?

> Beryllium

12

RHEUMATOLOGY

Arthropathies

Rheumatoid Arthritis (RA)

1331. In synovial fluid of a native joint, above what leukocyte count is an inflammatory etiology a likely diagnosis?

> 2,000

1332. In a patient with an underlying inflammatory disorder, how long does morning joint stiffness last?

> >1 hour

1333. Anti-CCP is specific for what diagnosis?

> RA

1334. In RA, is joint pain typically described as symmetric or asymmetric?

> Symmetric

1335. In the upper extremity, what joints does RA mainly affect? What is often seen on radiographs?

> MCP, PIP, wrists, and elbow

> Erosions, periarticular osteopenia and symmetric joint space narrowing

1336. In a patient with RA and arm paresthesias, what diagnosis should be considered?

> C1-C2 subluxation

1337. In a patient with RA and worsening hoarseness, what diagnosis should be considered?

> Cricoarytenoid involvement

1338. In a patient with RA and foot or wrist drop, what diagnosis should be considered?

> Mononeuritis multiplex

1339. What is the most common first-line disease modifying agent used in RA? What other medication should be started at the same time? What class of medications is added if symptoms continue to worsen?

> Methotrexate
> Folic acid
> Anti-TNF alpha medications

1340. What conditions should be screened for before starting Anti-TNF medications?

> Tuberculosis
> Hepatitis B and C

1341. Does methotrexate need to be discontinued in pregnancy? Why?

> Yes
> Teratogenic

Osteoarthritis (OA)

1342. What are Heberden and Bouchard nodes?

> Heberden: Bony swelling of the DIP joint
> Bouchard: Bony swelling of the PIP joint

1343. What is a Baker cyst?

> Popliteal synovial cyst
  - Commonly due to degenerative joint disease or other intraarticular pathology

1344. What is first line treatment for osteoarthritis?

> NSAIDs

1345. What non-pharmacologic intervention can be beneficial for knee and hip osteoarthritis?

> Weight loss

1346. Are opioids superior to non-opioid medications for osteoarthritis pain management?

> No

1347. When should surgical intervention be considered for severe osteoarthritis?

> ➤ Pain is no longer controlled with medications and/or injections
> ➤ Joint pain negatively effects activities of daily living

Hypertrophic Osteoarthropathy

1348. What is hypertrophic osteoarthropathy? What are the clinical features?

> ➤ Abnormal proliferation of skin and periosteal tissues involving the extremities
> ➤ Clinical features:
>   - Digital clubbing
>   - Periostosis of tubular bones
>   - Synovial effusions

1349. What comorbidities are associated with hypertrophic osteoarthropathy?

> ➤ Lung cancer, chronic pulmonary infections, COPD, and cardiac shunts

1350. How is pain associated with hypertrophic osteoarthropathy treated?

> ➤ Elevation of the involved limbs

Septic Arthropathy

1351. What synovial fluid leukocyte count is indicative of a septic arthropathy in a native joint? Prosthetic joint?

> ➤ Native: 50,000
> ➤ Prosthetic: 3,000

1352. Does the presence of crystals on synovial fluid analysis rule out a prosthetic joint infection?

> No, the two can occur concomitantly

1353. In septic arthritis, what is the classic physical exam finding?

> Severe joint pain that worsens with micromotion and passive flexion/extension

Crystalline Arthropathies

1354. What type of crystal deposition occurs with gout?

> Monosodium urate (MSU) crystals

1355. What is the "classic" location for gouty attacks? What is gout in this location called?

> First MTP joint
> Podagra

1356. Why are patients with heart failure more prone to gout flares?

> Diuresis can trigger gout

1357. How do monosodium urate crystals appear microscopically?

> Needle shaped with negative birefringence

1358. Does a normal uric acid level rule out an acute gout flare?

> No, uric acid levels can be falsely low during an acute flare

1359. What medication is the first line treatment for gout flares?

> NSAIDs

1360. What are considered second and third line medications for acute gout?
> Second: Colchicine
> Third: Steroids

1361. How soon after symptom onset should colchicine be initiated?
> Within 24 hours

1362. What is the first line preventative medication for gout?
> Allopurinol

1363. In Han Chinese, Taiwanese, and Korean patients with renal disease, what should be checked before starting allopurinol? Why?
> HLA B5801
> High risk for allergic reaction
  - Drug reaction with eosinophilia and systemic symptoms (DRESS) syndrome

1364. How should gouty cellulitis be treated? What should not be used?
> Prednisone
> Do not use antibiotics

1365. What medication should be used for severe recurrent or tophaceous gout not responding to standard therapy (i.e. allopurinol, febuxostat, probenecid)?
> Pegloticase

1366. What finding is present on x-ray in patients with asymptomatic calcium pyrophosphate deposition (CPPD)?
> Chondrocalcinosis

1367. What is seen microscopically in CPPD?

> Rhomboid shaped positively birefringent crystals

1368. In patients under 50 years old with CPPD, what 4 metabolic conditions should be screened for?

> **H**emochromatosis
> **H**ypomagnesemia
> **H**yperparathyroidism
> **H**ypothyroidism
>   ▪ Remember: "**4H**"

1369. What is first line systemic treatment for CPPD?

> NSAIDs

Seronegative Spondyloarthritides

1370. What four conditions are considered to be the spondyloarthritides?

> Psoriatic arthritis
> Reactive arthritis
> Ankylosing spondylitis (AS)
> IBD associated arthritis

1371. What serologic testing is often done, but is neither sensitive nor specific for spondyloarthritis?

> HLA-B27

1372. Sausage shaped fingers or toes and nail pitting is associated with what diagnosis?

> Psoriatic arthritis

1373. What is the first medication class used for psoriatic arthritis?

> NSAIDs

1374. If psoriatic arthritis is unresponsive to NSAIDs, what additional medication or medication classes can be prescribed?

> Methotrexate
> Anti-TNF medications

1375. What is the classic triad of reactive arthritis?

> **C**onjunctivitis
> U**R**ethritis
> **A**rthritis
  - Remember: "**C**lassic **R**eactive **A**rthritis"

1376. What infection must be evaluated for in a patient presenting with reactive arthritis?

> HIV

1377. What are the 5 most common pathogens that are thought to trigger reactive arthritis?

> Chlamydia trachomatis
> Yersinia
> Salmonella
> Shigella
> Campylobacter

1378. What is the treatment and prognosis for reactive arthritis?

> NSAIDs
  - May consider steroid injection if pain is severe
> Self-limited
  - Resolution may take several months

1379. What joints does AS typically involve?

> Sacroiliac
  - Commonly presents as bilateral sacroiliitis

1380. What are the classic symptoms of ankylosing spondylitis?

> Pain and stiffness that are worse with rest and improve with physical activity or heat

1381. What is the first imaging test that should be ordered for suspected ankylosing spondylitis?

> Spinal and pelvic x-rays

1382. What is seen on spinal and pelvic x-rays in patients with AS?

> Sclerosis, bony alkalosis (bamboo spine), pseudo-widening of joints, fusion of sacroiliac joints

1383. What is the first line treatment for AS?

> NSAIDs

1384. If AS symptoms are non-responsive to NSAIDs, what is the next medication class to consider?

> Anti-TNF agents

1385. In a patient with Crohn's disease presenting with polyarticular arthritis, what medication class can treat the underlying inflammatory bowel disease and prevent joint disease progression?

> Anti-TNF agent

Scleroderma

1386. What are the 3 classic skin findings in Scleroderma?

> Sclerodactyly
> Digital pitting
> Calcinosis

1387. How do skin findings vary between diffuse and limited cutaneous scleroderma (CREST syndrome)?

> ➤ Limited: Skin thickening typically proximal to the elbows and knees
> ➤ Diffuse: Involves the elbows, knees, and torso

1388. What antibodies can be used to differentiate limited and diffuse systemic sclerosis?

> ➤ Limited: Anticentromere
> ➤ Diffuse: Anti-SCL-70

1389. What primary pulmonary manifestations are seen in limited systemic sclerosis? Diffuse systemic sclerosis?

> ➤ Limited: Pulmonary hypertension
> ➤ Diffuse: Interstitial lung disease

1390. What is the primary cause of morbidity and mortality in patients with scleroderma?

> ➤ Pulmonary disease (ie. interstitial lung disease)

1391. What are the 4 typical presenting findings of scleroderma renal crisis?

> ➤ Hemolytic anemia
> ➤ Hypertension
> ➤ Thrombocytopenia
> ➤ Renal failure

1392. What is the first line treatment for scleroderma renal crisis?

> ➤ ACE Inhibitor
>   ▪ Even in setting of elevated creatinine

1393. What upper gastrointestinal finding is sometimes seen in patients with scleroderma and can result in chronic anemia?

> Gastric antral vascular ectasia (GAVE aka Watermelon stomach)

1394. What is the treatment for GAVE?

> Argon plasma coagulation (APC)

1395. What causes nephrogenic systemic fibrosis?

> Exposure to gadolinium in patients with renal failure (typically EGFR <30 mL/min/1.73m^2)

1396. Why are steroids minimized in scleroderma?

> Risk factor for precipitating scleroderma renal crisis

1397. What are the best non-pharmacologic methods to reduce the risk of Raynaud's phenomenon?

> Cold avoidance and maintenance of core temperature

> Smoking cessation

1398. What medications can be used for symptomatic Raynaud's phenomenon?

> Calcium channel blockers

> Sildenafil

> Nitroglycerin paste

1399. What two types of pulmonary hypertension can be caused by scleroderma?

> WHO I: From intrinsic pulmonary arterial hypertension

> WHO III: From intrinsic lung disease resulting in pulmonary hypertension

1400. What is first line treatment for patients with scleroderma associated ILD?

> Mycophenolate mofetil

Lupus

1401. In what disease is dsDNA positive, and how is it helpful in this setting?

> Systemic lupus erythematosus (SLE)
> Correlates with disease activity, especially renal involvement

1402. What is the classic rash seen in SLE?

> Malar "butterfly" rash

1403. On CMP and CBC, what lab abnormalities are seen in lupus?

> Elevated creatinine
> Pancytopenia (any one of the three cell lines may be low)
> Hypoalbuminemia

1404. What antibody is most commonly seen in lupus?

> ANA
> ▪ >95% sensitive, but not specific to lupus

1405. Does ANA titer correlate with disease activity?

> No

1406. What antibody is most commonly positive in drug-induced lupus?

> Anti-histone antibody

1407. What two medications are most commonly linked to drug associated lupus?

> Hydralazine
> Procainamide

1408. Other than dsDNA, what other antibody is specific to lupus?

> Anti-smith antibodies

1409. Other than dsDNA, what serologic marker can be checked to assess disease activity?
> C3 and C4
  - Commonly low when disease is active

1410. What clotting disorder is associated with lupus?
> Anti-phospholipid antibody syndrome (APLS)

1411. What medication is continued indefinitely in most patients with lupus? Why?
> Hydroxychloroquine
> Reduces flares

1412. What screening exam should be done annually in patients on hydroxychloroquine?
> Ophthalmologic exam

1413. What medication, along with prednisone, is considered first line treatment for patients with lupus nephritis?
> Mycophenolate mofetil

1414. What 3 medications are typically used as first line agents in patients with life-threatening disease manifestations?
> High dose steroids
> Cyclophosphamide
> Mycophenolate mofetil

1415. What is Libman-Sacks endocarditis?
> Nonbacterial thrombotic endocarditis
  - Often seen in patient with SLE and positive antiphospholipid antibodies
  - Not correlated with disease activity

Myositis

1416. What physical exam finding is classically seen in patients with myositis?

> Proximal muscle weakness

1417. What 3 dermatologic findings are seen in dermatomyositis?

> Gottron papules: Scaly purple papules/plaques overlying joints

> Heliotrope rash: Lilac discoloration of periorbital tissue, with or without edema

> Mechanic's hands: Uncomfortable fissuring and scaling of the lateral surfaces of the fingers

1418. In a patient diagnosed with dermatomyositis, what else should they be evaluated for?

> Underlying malignancy
  - Ensure age appropriate cancer screening is up to date

1419. What is first line treatment for myositis?

> High dose steroids

1420. When evaluating a patient for myopathy, what other etiologies should be considered other than inflammatory?

> Thyroid mediated myopathy

> Steroid mediated (exogenous or endogenous) myopathy

> Statin mediated direct muscle injury

1421. How is inclusion body myositis characterized?

> Insidious onset involving proximal and distal muscles, including the finger flexors

> Asymmetric distribution

1422. What antibody is often present in statin-associated necrotizing autoimmune myositis?

> Anti-HMG Co-A reductase

1423. What antibody is commonly positive in antisynthetase syndrome?

> Anti-Jo-1

Muscular Pain & Weakness

Fibromyalgia

1424. What are the characteristic symptoms of fibromyalgia?

> Global pain
> Fatigue and disrupted sleep
> Exercise intolerance

1425. What are the hallmark lab findings in fibromyalgia?

> Normal CBC, BMP, TSH, and ESR/CRP

1426. What are the first line non-pharmacologic treatments for fibromyalgia?

> Aerobic exercise
> Cognitive behavioral therapy

1427. What medications have been approved for the treatment of fibromyalgia?

> Duloxetine
> Pregabalin
> Milnacipran

Polymyalgia Rheumatica (PMR)

1428. In a patient with proximal muscle tenderness and an inability to brush their own hair, what diagnosis should be suspected?

> ➢ PMR

1429. What lab value is usually elevated in PMR?

> ➢ ESR
>> ▪ Mild to moderate elevation, as compared to a severe elevation in giant cell arteritis

1430. What is the treatment for PMR?

> ➢ Low dose steroids

Vasculitis

Large Vessel Vasculitis

1431. What are the two most common types of large vessel vasculitis?

> ➢ Giant cell arteritis
> ➢ Takayasu arteritis

1432. What is the characteristic age and presentation for patient with GCA?

> ➢ Age >50 years old
> ➢ Headaches, scalp tenderness, jaw claudication, visual changes

1433. How is the diagnosis of GCA confirmed?

> ➢ Temporal artery biopsy

1434. What is treatment for GCA?

> ➢ High dose steroids
>> ▪ Do not wait for biopsy scheduling or results

1435. What is the general age for patients with Takayasu arteritis?

> ➢ ~30 years old
>> ▪ Younger than GCA

1436. What are the common presenting symptoms in a patient with Takayasu arteritis?

> ➢ Extremity claudication
> ➢ Pulse deficits
> ➢ Asymmetric brachial blood pressure readings

Small & Medium Vessel Vasculitis

1437. What medium vessel vasculitis is associated with hepatitis B infections?

> ➢ Polyarteritis Nodosa

1438. What three parts of the body are classically involved in granulomatosis with polyangiitis (GPA)?

> ➢ Sinuses: Sinusitis
> ➢ Lungs: Pulmonary infiltrates, cavitary lesions, or hemorrhage
> ➢ Kidneys: Renal failure (ie. pauci-immune glomerulonephritis)
>> ▪ No complement or IgG/A/M on DIF

1439. What serology is positive in GPA?

> ➢ C-ANCA (anti-PR3)

1440. What is the treatment for GPA?

> ➢ High dose steroids
> ➢ Cyclophosphamide or rituximab
> ➢ Plasma exchange if organ/life threatening disease is present

- PEXIVAS study (2021) did not show an added benefit of plasma exchange

1441. How does microscopic polyangiitis differ from GPA clinically?

  ➢ Palpable purpura can be present
  ➢ Sinuses are rarely affected

1442. What serology is positive in microscopic polyangiitis?

  ➢ P-ANCA (anti-MPO)

1443. What are the characteristic findings in eosinophilic granulomatosis with polyangiitis (EGPA)?

  ➢ Asthma
  ➢ Eosinophilia
  ➢ Elevated IgE
  ➢ Pulmonary involvement

1444. What antibody is positive in EGPA?

  ➢ P-ANCA (anti-MPO)

1445. In which age group is Henoch-Schonlein purpura (HSP) typically diagnosed?

  ➢ Children

1446. HSP typically involves which parts of the body?

  ➢ Skin: Palpable purpura
  ➢ Joint: Arthritis
  ➢ GI: Abdominal pain
  ➢ Kidney: Glomerulonephritis

1447. What infection is associated with cryoglobulinemic vasculitis?

  ➢ Hepatitis C

1448. In what country is Behçet's syndrome most common?

> Turkey

1449. What are the typical symptoms of Behçet's syndrome?

> Oral and genital ulcers
> Uveitis
> Rashes (ie. erythema nodosum, pseudofolliculitis)
> Asymmetric oligoarthritis

1450. What vasculitis affects small to medium sized vessels in cigarette smokers?

> Thromboangiitis obliterans

1451. How does primary angiitis of the CNS present?

> Recurrent headaches
> Stroke, TIA
> Encephalopathy

1452. How is primary angiitis of the CNS diagnosed?

> Lumbar puncture: Lymphocytic pleocytosis and elevated protein
  - Brain biopsy often falsely negative because of patchy distribution
  - Serum inflammatory markers often normal
> Need high index of suspicion

1453. How is primary angiitis of the CNS treated?

> High dose steroids
> Cyclophosphamide

1454. In Kawasaki disease, what is the greatest predictor for long term cardiovascular events?

> Persistence of coronary artery aneurysm

Bone Health

1455. In what condition can bisphosphonates be useful for pain, even in the absence of osteoporosis?

> Complex regional pain syndrome

1456. What is the difference between a T-score and a Z-score?

> T-score compares bone density to that of a healthy sex matched 30 year old
> Z-score compares to age and sex matched controls

1457. How is osteoporosis diagnosed in postmenopausal women?

> DEXA scan T-score <-2.5

1458. What is first line treatment for osteoporosis?

> Bisphosphonates

1459. What are the two main adverse effects of bisphosphonates that should be monitored for?

> Pill esophagitis
> Osteonecrosis of the jaw
>   ▪ Rare, tends to occur in immunocompromised patients

1460. In osteoporosis, what happens to the serum levels of calcium, phosphorous, alkaline phosphatase and PTH?

> All normal

1461. What is the primary vitamin deficiency in osteomalacia and rickets?

> Vitamin D deficiency

1462. What is the pathophysiology of Paget's disease of bone?

➢ Abnormally rapid bone destruction (osteoclasts) and reformation (osteoblasts)

1463. Paget's disease is a risk factor for what malignancy?

➢ Osteosarcoma

1464. What medications can put patients at risk for bony avascular necrosis?

➢ High dose steroids

Sjogren Syndrome

1465. What are the 3 common characteristics of Sjogren Syndrome?

➢ Keratoconjunctivitis sicca
➢ Xerostomia
➢ Salivary gland enlargement

1466. What two antibodies are commonly positive in Sjogren Syndrome?

➢ Anti-Ro (SSA)
➢ Anti-La (SSB)

1467. What malignancy are patients with Sjogren syndrome at increased risk for?

➢ B-cell lymphoma

Miscellaneous

1468. Anti-smooth muscle antibody is specific for what autoimmune diagnosis?

➢ Autoimmune hepatitis

1469. Mixed connective tissue disease (MCTD) is a diagnosis consisting of at least 2 of what three rheumatologic conditions?

> SLE
> Scleroderma
> Polymyositis

1470. What antibody is present in MCTD?

> Anti-U1-RNP antibodies

1471. In MCTD, what is the most common etiology of mortality?

> Pulmonary hypertension

1472. In a patient who gets recurrent red, hot painful ears, what diagnosis should be considered?

> Relapsing polychondritis

1473. What findings are typical in familial Mediterranean fever (FMF)?

> Recurrent, self-limited fevers that begin during childhood or adolescence
> Serositis
> Arthritis
> Self-limited rashes

1474. What is first line treatment for FMF?

> Colchicine
  - Prevents attacks and development of AA amyloidosis

1475. What are the classic symptoms for adult-onset Still's disease?

> Fever
> Evanescent rash
  - "Salmon colored"

> Inflammatory arthritis

1476. What lab marker is profoundly elevated in adult-onset Still's disease?

> Ferritin (>2,500 μg/L)

1477. For adult-onset Still's disease refractory to steroids, what other medications can be considered?

> Anakinra
> Tocilizumab

1478. In pemphigus vulgaris, what component of the epithelium is the target of antibodies?

> Desmoglein
  ▪ Found in desmosomes

1479. In bullous pemphigoid, what is the target of autoantibodies?

> Hemidesmosomes

Rheumatology

13

SLEEP

Obstructive Sleep Apnea & Obesity Hypoventilation Syndrome

1480. What are characteristic symptoms of obstructive sleep apnea (OSA)?

> ➢ Snoring
> ➢ Apnea
> ➢ Excessive daytime sleepiness
> ➢ Morning headache

1481. What are characteristic physical exam findings for patients with OSA or suspected OSA?

> ➢ Obesity
> ➢ Enlarged soft palate
> ➢ Neck circumference ≥16 inches (women) or ≥17 inches (men)

1482. What is the biggest risk factor for OSA?

> ➢ Obesity, especially with adipose tissue in truck or neck

1483. During the day, what is the PaO2 for a patient with OSA (low, normal, or high)?

> ➢ Normal

1484. On a sleep study, the severity of OSA is classified by what index?

> ➢ Apnea-hypopnea index (AHI): Number of apneas plus hypopneas per hour of sleep

1485. What AHI threshold is diagnostic of OSA on a sleep apnea?

> ➢ AHI ≥5 per hour

1486. What patients can be considered for home sleep testing?

> High pretest probability of moderate to severe uncomplicated OSA (ie. no significant comorbidities like COPD, HF, neuromuscular weakness, stroke)

1487. What is the treatment of choice in OSA? What symptom is the strongest indication for this treatment?

> Continuous positive airway pressure (CPAP)
> Excessive daytime sleepiness

1488. What should be done for a patient recently started on a CPAP for OSA that endorses sore throat and nasal congestion?

> In-line humidification (upper airway symptoms are common side effect of CPAP)

1489. When should surgery be considered for OSA?

> In patients who do not improve with CPAP or refuse CPAP (surgery is NOT first line treatment)

1490. What does a daytime ABG show for a patient with obesity hypoventilation syndrome (OHS)?

> Decreased PaO2, increase PaCO2 (>45 mmHg)

1491. What cardiac complications can result from untreated OHS?

> Biventricular failure
> Pulmonary hypertension

Central Sleep Apnea

1492. What is central sleep apnea?

> Lack of respiratory effort due to decreased ventilatory drive from the brain

1493. What is the classic ventilation pattern seen in heart failure due to central sleep apnea?
> Cheyne-Stokes breathing: Crescendo-decrescendo pattern of ventilation

1494. For a patient with heart failure and Cheynes-Stokes breathing pattern, what is the best treatment?
> Further diuresis and optimization of heart failure regimen

1495. What cardiac comorbidity, other than heart failure, is a risk factor for central sleep apnea?
> Atrial fibrillation

Narcolepsy

1496. What symptoms are characteristic of narcolepsy?
> Daytime sleepiness
> Cataplexy (emotionally triggered transient muscle weakness)
> Hypnagogic hallucinations: Vivid hallucinations while falling asleep
> Sleep paralysis: Inability to move 1-2 minutes after awakening

1497. What is the most common first line pharmacologic treatment for daytime sleepiness in narcolepsy?
> Modafinil

Miscellaneous

1498. What should be screened for and treated, if present, in a patient with restless leg syndrome?

➢ Iron deficiency

1499. What is the diagnosis of someone who works the night shift but reports >6 months of excessive sleepiness and neurocognitive dysfunction when awake?

➢ Shift work sleep disorder

1500. In a patient with excessive daytime sleepiness who is not able to give an accurate sleep diary, what is the next step?

➢ Actigraphy

Notes

Notes

Notes

Notes